7·30 - 9·00.
5 - 7·30.
Fri. 9 - 12.

2¹² ,
$$\frac{3}{6}$$

NURSING THE AGED

Edited by *Pat Young*
Editor-in-Chief, Geriatric Medicine

Woodhead-Faulkner · Cambridge

Published by Woodhead-Faulkner Ltd
Fitzwilliam House, 32 Trumpington Street, Cambridge CB2 1QY

First published 1984
© Pat Young 1984
ISBN (Paper) 0 85941 244 X
ISBN (Cased) 0 85941 242 3

Library of Congress Cataloging in Publication Data

Nursing the aged.

Includes index.
1. Geriatric nursing. I. Young, Pat.
[DNLM: 1. Geriatric Nursing. WY 152 N9795]
RC954.N893   1984   610.73'65   84–13190
ISBN 0–85941–242–3
ISBN 0–85941–244–X (pbk.)

Designed by Geoff Green
Typeset by Wyvern Typesetting Limited, Bristol
Printed in Great Britain by
St Edmundsbury Press, Bury St Edmunds, Suffolk

PREFACE

I would like to take this opportunity to express my warm appreciation to each author who has contributed to this book and, in particular, to Ruth Manley for her additional help and advice. Everyone has risen to the challenge of writing for a wide and diverse readership with enthusiasm and skill, and the book shows, if nothing else, how true it is that geriatric care is a matter of teamwork, and that all those involved are deeply committed to their task. It has been a great pleasure and privilege for me to work with such a distinguished team of authors, each one an acknowledged expert in his or her own field.

I would also like to thank Mrs Ann Meyer, Nursing Officer, and Miss Lynn Price, Ward Sister, All Saints' Hospital, Eastbourne, for sparing the time to read the manuscript and to make useful comments and suggestions, and the publishers, for their continued encouragement and confidence in the book during its gestation and birth.

Throughout the text, in order to distinguish easily between them, the patient is referred to as male, and the nurse or carer, as female, although their genders are obviously interchangeable. Drugs are referred to by their generic names only, as it would have been impossible to give a comprehensive and up-to-date list of all the proprietary brands available.

Lastly, I would like to dedicate this book to my dear uncle, Mr F. C. Ross, who became my guardian after my parents' death, and who, at the age of 89, is a living example of the dignity, wisdom, and experience which only come with age, and which we should all honour and respect far more than we do. I owe him more than I can ever say.

I sincerely hope readers will find this book useful, and I shall welcome their suggestions for its improvement for future editions.

Pat Young
March 1984

CONTENTS

INTRODUCTION

PAT YOUNG

Editor-in-Chief, Geriatric Medicine

It is a truism that old age will come to all of us if we are lucky – or unlucky, depending on the circumstances in which we end our lives. Those of us who are lucky will have loving families to cherish and care for us; those less fortunate will end their days in some kind of institution.

Statistics show that there will be an enormous increase in the ageing population over the next 20 years, particularly in those aged over 75, who will suffer most from illness, or some sort of disability. They will need care – whether at home, in hospital or in residential care – and the burden will fall increasingly heavily on nurses, nursing auxiliaries, care assistants, voluntary workers and relatives.

This book is intended to help anyone who may be involved in nursing the aged, by offering information and guidance of an essentially practical nature. It is not an academic text, but a practical handbook, which I hope can be read with profit by trained nurses and untrained relatives alike. The author of each chapter has been asked to present his or her material in a style which can be understood by any intelligent adult, but at the same time to make no concessions to the lay reader at the expense of the trained nurse. This has been no easy task, but the 9 authors have all risen to the challenge nobly, and I hope you will find the result of their efforts worth while.

In this introduction, and before the experts take over, I would like to discuss the special qualities and approach that nursing the aged demands. Far too many distressing stories are told about the misery and degradation suffered by elderly patients to dismiss this as unnecessary. Examples are quoted constantly in both the lay and the nursing press and, as recently as May 1983, an observation study of elderly people in four different care environments was published under the title *Time for Action*, by the University of Sheffield Joint Unit for Social Services Research, which described many scenes in which old people were subjected to indignities by the so-called 'caring' staff.

While nurses are under considerable pressure in this exacting branch of their profession, this does not absolve them from treating elderly patients as inanimate objects. Examples quoted in this study include shaving a female patient's face with an electric razor in the middle of the lounge; putting an old lady's lunch plate on top of her folded hands, without looking to see that the table top was clear; wheeling an old lady from the bathroom to her bed on a hoist with her bare buttocks hanging through the commode-type seat, exposing her anus; changing a patient's knickers, without pulling the curtains around her bed; and talking about a patient in front of her as if she wasn't there, or couldn't understand what was being said. Perhaps one of the greatest humiliations an old person can suffer is to be incontinent and unable to reach the toilet in time. This study also quotes cases of patients not being allowed, or helped, to go to the toilet when they asked, or being made to walk to the toilet when they asked for a wheelchair.

These may seem trivial offences against a person's dignity but when that person is old, confused, ill and vulnerable, they can cause unnecessary additional suffering. And they are sufficiently typical of a general attitude towards the aged to be very worrying. There is no doubt that very old people, especially if they are handicapped in some way, or confused or demented, can be extremely difficult to handle. So can children, but, because they are in the all-important formative years, with their lives before them, they command far more public sympathy and concern for their welfare, both in hospital and out of it, than those at the other end of the age scale. We tend to draw back from the elderly and to see in them an unwelcome picture of ourselves in 20 or 30 years' time which we cannot – or will not – face. Perhaps we are protecting our own sensitivities by adopting an unfeeling, even callous, attitude towards them, but this is still no excuse for causing them discomfort and misery.

It is an accepted cliché that geriatrics is an unpopular specialty in medicine. Certainly this was true some 20 years ago when it attracted only those doctors who saw it as a quick road to promotion, or who couldn't get a job in any other specialty, but now the younger generation of doctors specialising in geriatric medicine is of a noticeably higher calibre. They evidently see the challenge in this rapidly expanding field and the scope it offers to practise their skills.

Nurses, too, have been reluctant to work in a geriatric hospital or unit, seeing their task as hard and unrewarding. But often, after an enforced period on a geriatric ward, many become so committed to their elderly patients that they do not want to work anywhere else, and apply enthusiastically for places on courses in geriatric nursing.

Nursing the aged demands true tender, loving care. As one ward sister in a geriatric hospital said to me: 'You have to think of them as your mother or father. You mustn't be afraid of putting your arms round them and loving them, if you think they need it.' Her ward, which has been imaginatively upgraded, has more the atmosphere of a comfortable, well run, homely hotel, where the interests and well-being of the guests are paramount, than of a medical institution where the patients are subjugated to the discipline and authority of the staff.

So good nursing care for the aged is possible and certainly is practised. It requires vision and sensitivity, compassion and concern, infinite patience and a deep understanding of what it is like to be old. The old, after all, are only our future selves. They are the same people they always were but their bodies, and sometimes their minds, don't function as well as they used to, and they have to suffer all the consequent frustrations and difficulties. The old need sympathy and support, as well as respect for the dignity of their years and experience. Wisdom, which only comes with age, is a quality much undervalued in today's society.

Our whole society has got to take a different attitude towards ageing. The words 'old' and 'geriatric' must no longer be used as offensive epithets. We have got to start valuing and respecting our older generation again – as is done in many other countries considered 'less civilised' than ours. In the People's Republic of China, for instance, it is written into the constitution that children must look after their parents in old age. Grandparents are an important part of the family unit. Their function is to run the household, help in the local community, and to look after their grandchildren in order that their own children can go out to work. I led a group of nurses on a study tour of the health services in China in 1978. As the party included a matron of an old people's home and a nursing sister of a geriatric ward, we asked if we could visit the equivalent Chinese institutions. Our Chinese guides were at a loss to understand what we meant, as such homes do not exist there. They were horrified to learn how we treat our old folk.

The essence of good nursing care for the aged, therefore, springs from an innate respect. This emerges powerfully from a handbook of guidelines, called *Improving Geriatric Care in Hospital*, which was produced jointly by the British Geriatrics Society and the Royal College of Nursing in 1975. These two organisations, with the support of the Department of Health and Social Security, were so concerned by the low standards of nursing care in geriatric wards and hospitals that they set up a working group to find out why and where standards were falling short, and to prepare guidelines that would help to improve matters. These guidelines were published, and have been used as the basis of a teaching package for hospital staff and for anyone nursing the elderly.

The results of the survey carried out by this working group showed that there were four main areas where nursing care of older patients was generally poor. First, and possibly most important, their feelings were not considered, and their dignity, privacy and sense of personal identity were not maintained. Second, they were neither allowed nor encouraged to be independent and to perform small tasks for themselves; nor to be mobile. They were too often kept in bed or in a chair because there they would be less of a nuisance to nursing staff. Third, not enough attention was given to their personal hygiene or physiological needs (this shortcoming mainly concerned those patients who were incontinent). Fourth, they were not offered enough social or recreational activity to make life more bearable.

Of course things were not bad everywhere, but so many hospitals were short of nursing staff that the sheer pressure of work often meant that they didn't have time to do more than the basic nursing tasks, and sometimes these had to be skimped. There certainly wasn't enough time to stop and talk to patients, let alone time to stop and think what could be done to make their lives easier. There is a lesson here: where the very young and the very old are concerned (both being so helpless and vulnerable when ill), taking the time to give them real tender, loving care is vitally important. Consideration, understanding, respect and affection are essential to their well-being and can make all the difference, not only to their comfort but also to their recovery.

So what is the right approach to take? Let us look at the four areas of care where faults may lie, see where the approach is wrong, and how we can avoid making the same mistakes ourselves.

DIGNITY, PRIVACY AND PERSONAL IDENTITY

Do you react as resentfully as I do to being called 'dear' by a total stranger, particularly if he or she is performing a service? Perhaps I am touchy, but I find it unnecessarily familiar and patronising. I don't see why people can't say 'Madam', if they do not know my name. A good nurse will never call a patient 'dear', or by a Christian or pet name, unless a good personal relationship has been established and the patient has given express permission. An elderly patient should never be called 'Gran' or 'Dad'. The patient's surname and correct title – Mr, Mrs or Miss – should always be used until such time as the relationship develops to allow a more informal approach. This is what dignity is all about – being treated as a person with some status in the world and whose feelings matter. The old, who no longer have the status of a job and the income that goes with it, often lack the respect they should command, and this is only too true in many hospitals where busy staff rely on the ubiquitous word 'dear' rather than take time to remember and use each individual's proper name.

Think how daunting it must be for a sick, elderly person to have to come into the noise and bustle of a busy ward, to cope with a totally strange and rather forbidding environment, to adjust to the necessary discipline of an institution and to surrender – body and soul – to the care of strangers. If a patient is received in an offhand manner, and treated as a 'case' undeserving of respect or consideration, his confusion and apprehension will be magnified and he will feel disorientated and miserable. What a difference it will make to him to be met with courtesy and kindness, to be shown his bed and where to put his belongings, to have the ward routine explained and to be introduced to the other patients and staff. At once his fears will begin to subside – instead of being nervous and defensive he will become relaxed and co-operative, thus making the nurse's job much easier.

Privacy is especially important to an old person, who is likely to be shy, modest and embarrassed over those functions of daily living that he normally performs in private, such as washing, dressing, undressing and going to the toilet. In a ward the nurse should always draw the curtains around a patient's bed when intimate procedures are being carried out, particularly if a urinal, bedpan or commode is being used. If the patient is able to use the toilet, the door should never be left wide open so that he can be seen by anyone passing.

With a continually shifting patient population in hospitals, it is only too easy for personal identities to become submerged when the medical and nursing staff tend to think of 'the fractured neck of femur in bed 4' rather than of Mrs Bloggins from Hackney. Patients should always be thought of, and treated, as individual human beings, not as cases, and the first step towards preserving a patient's identity is to mark his bed, locker and belongings with his name, initials and title, and to refer to him by his name. An effort should be made to get to know the patient and something of his life and background, and to establish a rapport and a good working relationship with him, which will be helpful to both throughout the period of illness or hospitalisation. A patient's personality and experience of life may have a considerable effect on his behaviour and response to treatment.

There is still an unfortunate tendency for doctors on a ward round, or nurses making beds, to talk to each other over a patient's head, as if he wasn't there, and this is all the more discourteous if they are talking about him. Of course, this is something *you* would never do! Old people, who may be a bit deaf or a little confused, are especially vulnerable to this sort of behaviour and it must make them feel even more isolated and anxious than they do already.

There is also a tendency to treat elderly patients like children. Even though some of them do behave like children, there is no excuse for making them wear bibs if they dribble or eat messily, and for telling them they are 'naughty' if they wet the bed, or to 'eat up your nice milk pudding because it's good for you', if they leave it untouched. Perhaps they detest milk pudding, and they certainly don't wet the bed on purpose, so their shame and discomfort will be compounded by being made to feel guilty or a nuisance. Try to put yourself in the patient's place, and never assume that he doesn't have feelings just because he can't communicate them.

INDEPENDENCE AND MOBILITY

The days are long gone when it was thought best to keep patients in bed all day when they were ill, and when older patients were not expected to recover to live an active life again. Nowadays the accent is on rehabilitation, and it is the aim of all good departments of geriatric medicine to help their patients to get up and about again as soon as possible, and to return home to live a reasonably active and independent life. However, it is second nature for nurses to care for others and sometimes they may be misled by their generous instincts into doing too much for their patients, when it would be better to encourage them to do things for themselves. It is a mistake, for instance, to be over-protective of a stroke patient who has lost the use of one arm, and may also have difficulty with walking and with his speech. It may seem hard-hearted, but it will help him far more in the long run if he is encouraged to use his remaining powers and develop his capabilities as much as possible. He will then not fall into the habit of depending on others, but will become self-reliant to some extent, and this will boost his morale considerably. There is nothing more demoralising for an active person than not to be able to do things for himself.

In hospital, a physiotherapist will give older patients simple exercises, both active and passive, to keep their joints mobile and to restore muscle function. She will teach them how to walk again, using whatever aid she considers necessary, such as crutches, a walking frame or a stick. (This is described in detail in chapter 9.) Physiotherapists are not always available round the clock in hospitals, and home visiting services are still limited, so it is the nurse's important task to see that the patient continues to do the exercises given by the physiotherapist, in order that he gets the full benefit from them and makes progress. It is equally important for a district nurse to see that exercises are done at home and to teach the patient's relatives to supervise them.

However, with a very sick, old person, there may well come a time when his physical abilities decline steadily and he needs help to perform all natural functions. This is where good nursing – real tender loving care – comes into its own. One point to remember if the patient is restless and confused: he or she should not be restrained by high cot-sides or by a chair tray, for example, unless the need to do so has been fully discussed and decided upon by the medical and nursing staff caring for that patient. A restraining harness should not be used under any circumstances.

PERSONAL HYGIENE AND PHYSIOLOGICAL NEEDS

Most old people wear dentures and many need spectacles and hearing aids. It goes without saying that these aids should be kept scrupulously clean and in good working order. Where dentures are concerned, if these are taken away from the bedside for cleaning, they should be marked carefully so that they don't get lost or mixed up with other patients' dentures. Materials are now available for marking dentures, but, if they are not to hand, their container should be clearly marked with the patient's name, and care taken that only his dentures are kept in it. Personal cleanliness is very important, of course, both for a patient in hospital or being nursed at home. Besides regular washing and bathing, patients should be encouraged and helped to take an interest in their personal appearance. Men should be encouraged to use the barber, and ladies, the hairdresser (if one is available). Ladies' facial hair (which increases with age) should be removed in privacy. Patients should be allowed to wear their own clothes, if possible, not those supplied by the hospital. These should be kept clean and in good order. It must be demoralising to have your clothes taken away from you and to be made to wear institutional garments which have been worn by other people, just because it is easier for the nurses who have to cope with the laundry service. This is one of the things that deprives a patient of his personal identity and dignity.

Another contributory factor is being incontinent – suffering the humiliation and indignity of wetting or soiling the bed or one's clothing, because the bladder or sphincter can no longer be controlled properly. There are many causes of incontinence in the elderly (these are described in chapter 2) but it is salutary to remember that it may be caused by the actions of nursing staff. Here is a typical example.

> A shy, nervous old lady was admitted to hospital with bronchitis, and was placed in a bed far away from the toilet. No one took the trouble to tell her where it was. Someone had put cot-sides on her bed, although she was not restless. In the middle of the night, when she needed to use the toilet, she had to climb over the end of the bed, and fell and hurt her knee. The nurses were busy at the other end of ward and no one noticed what had happened, so she had to get herself back into bed where, in her distress, she passed urine. She lay there crying in shame and from the pain of her injured knee. A nurse heard her eventually and came, all brusque efficiency, to see what was the matter. When she lifted

the bedclothes to examine the knee, she saw the bed was wet, and was obviously put out at having to fetch clean sheets and remake the bed. The old lady certainly got no sympathy from her.

The next morning the old lady's knee was too sore for her to walk, and, not wanting to make a fuss, she said she didn't want to go when the nurse came to take her to the toilet. No one offered her a bedpan and she was too shy to ask. The inevitable eventually happened; she wet the bed again. This time, however, the nurse on duty was tactful and concerned. She saw how painful the old lady's knee was and called the doctor to examine it. She put a commode beside her bed after she had wheeled her to the bathroom and washed her. The old lady was much more comfortable and her 'incontinence' vanished.

It is essential with older patients whose bladder or sphincter control is poor to make sure that they have easy access to a toilet or commode if they can get up. If not, a bedpan or urinal should be offered to them at regular and frequent intervals. Incontinent patients should *never* be left sitting on a waterproof sheet without their undergarments or pyjama trousers. There are plenty of protective pads, pants and other appliances available. To be incontinent is the ultimate indignity, and a good nurse will do all she can to relieve the patient's discomfort.

SOCIAL NEEDS

We need just as much social contact and diversion towards the end of our lives as we do earlier on – perhaps more, as there is little else, other than meal times, to occupy our time. Whether in hospital, an old people's home, a nursing home or in his own home, a sick or disabled old person needs to see his family and friends often, to have the company of a beloved pet, to have his cherished belongings around him and to enjoy some form of entertainment or interest. Watching television from one end of the day to the other is *not* the answer!

Occupational therapists who work with the elderly have much to contribute here, as Anne Dummett describes in chapter 10. The confused or demented elderly present a particular problem, but methods are being developed of capturing their wandering thoughts and bringing them back to the realities of everyday life. This is called 'reality orientation' – a simple technique practised successfully in many geriatric and psychogeriatric hospitals and units.

Old people's minds can be stimulated also by memories of past events, by old songs or melodies they knew and loved when they were young, by pictures of historic occasions, such as royal jubilees, weddings and coronations, and by photographs of people, places and events that remind them of their youth. It is good to encourage old people to reminisce about their past lives – good for them and good for us too, for we may learn things of great interest and value.

Anyone who is nursing an elderly person needs first of all to know something about the condition from which he is suffering, what treatment he is being given, how he is likely to react to it, what progress can be expected and what the probable outcome will be. The early chapters in this book, written by doctors, supply this knowledge and explain how an older person reacts differently from young people as his physical and mental functions change with age. First, a consultant in geriatric medicine explains how the ageing process affects the body and gives detailed information about the conditions and diseases that are most common in the older generation. A psychiatrist who specialises in care of the elderly (a psychogeriatrician) describes their mental and psychological disorders and how they can be treated. A chapter is devoted to drug therapy because it is vitally important to understand how and why older people react differently to certain drugs, and to realise that they may have problems that other people do not have. For example, an old person is likely to have two or three things wrong with him at the same time, so those who are caring for him must be careful that the drugs he is given do not conflict with each other and produce side-effects that are worse than the disease itself. There is the added difficulty of making sure that someone who may be confused, or whose sight and hearing are not good, takes the right drugs in the right doses at the right time.

The chapters that follow are the core of this book. Written by nurses, they describe the specialised nursing care appropriate to an elderly patient, and are based on the famous definition of nursing given by the eminent American nurse, Virginia Henderson, who stated that nursing was helping a patient to perform those routine functions of daily living that he would normally perform himself. Eating, sleeping, washing, dressing, eliminating waste products from the body, communicating with other people – these are all things we perform for ourselves without a second thought, but when we are ill or disabled we may not be able to, and need someone's help. That someone is usually a nurse. Dying, too, is a part of life, and the nursing section ends with a sensitively written chapter on nursing care of the dying.

Doctors and nurses who work with the elderly have the support of other professionals who have special skills and specialised roles to play. They include physiotherapists, occupational therapists and dietitians, and there is a chapter from a member of each of these professions, describing the work they do and how it helps patients. The book ends with a brief survey of the services offered by social workers and by various voluntary organisations which provide practical help and support to those caring for handicapped or ill old people.

'An old man loved is winter with flowers.' This is an old German proverb which could be applied to nursing the aged. I hope this book will help all those who read it to plant a few flowers in the bleak landscape of their aged patients' lives.

Further reading

Improving Geriatric Care in Hospital: Report of a working party of the British Geriatrics Society and the Royal College of Nursing of the United Kingdom (The Royal College of Nursing, Henrietta Place, London W1M 0AB, 1975).

Godlove, Caroline; Richard, Lesley; and Rodwell, Graham, *Time for Action: An observation study of elderly people in four different care environments* (The Joint Unit for Social Services Research, University of Sheffield, 1983).

1

THE AGEING PROCESS

DR W. B. WRIGHT

Consultant in Geriatric Medicine,
Querns Hospital, Cirencester

It is natural to die in old age. Because of this, and because every one of us has had dealings with an invalid old person at some time or other, it is easy to see old age through pessimistic eyes. This pessimism does not affect the laity only. Some young nurses and doctors can leave the best training schools in Britain with a very dim view of the specialty of 'geriatrics' and all that it entails. Teaching centres are still orientated far too positively towards 'cure' rather than 'care'. The teachers still tend to throw up their hands helplessly when confronted with an invalid old person, almost as if diagnosis was an academic exercise, and treatment irrelevant. This is quite unfair to the elderly. It is an assumption that all their ills are irreversibly degenerative, as if they were immune to all the other types of illness, treatable or not, to which mankind is prone. The majority of elderly people, though they must die, will not spend years of invalidism before their end. For most of us, the end comes quietly and gently. For every old person you can think of who has died a chronic invalid there will have been at least four others who left this world after less than a month's illness.

Much can be done to anticipate and prevent disability among the elderly who are becoming invalid and, in some cases, to reverse it. All elderly people become frail in many respects. This should not interfere with their ability to lead a good life. They will have less muscular strength, and be unable to climb several flights of stairs readily, but they can expect to feel well and to be able to get about as much as they feel inclined to do, at least indoors. Their eyesight becomes impaired, as does their hearing, but, given appropriate aids, some reading and listening should be possible. There is always some recent memory loss which affects the learning ability, but, by the time this happens, most old people are settled into a way of living which makes these defects hardly noticeable.

The elderly, like the middle-aged, have a characteristic shape – the old person's stoop is as identifiable as middle-aged spread and height is always lost to some extent owing to degenerative changes in the spine and intervertebral discs. The aching and creaking of osteoarthritic joints is universal as age advances. Slackening joint ligaments bring changes in the hands and feet, particularly the latter, as a result of which fallen arches, corns and bunions become more prevalent. Those areas of skin which have been exposed to the sunlight throughout life, wrinkle and dis-colour. Nails may become dry and brittle, and difficulty in bending may make it impossible for old people to pare their toenails independently, which can result in ugly talons (onychogryphosis). Head hair becomes thinner, though facial hair is often coarser. Paradoxically, hair in the nostrils and ears may grow excessively. These surface changes make it increasingly important for elderly people to devote extra time to their appearance. Degeneration of the teeth and gums is inevitable, but good dental hygiene and appropriate dentures help a lot.

Apart from these universal changes, the elderly have diminished reserves with which to face encroaching illness. Once the internal environment has been assaulted, restoration of the normal state is more difficult and takes longer. These differences are evident from middle age onwards and some will now be considered in more detail.

FLUID BALANCE

The importance of this aspect of physiology for the elderly must be appreciated. To do this it is worth returning to first principles briefly. Man is descended from a sea creature. Within the confines of our waterproof skin we carry over 40 litres of water, the equivalent of more than three stacked crates of litre bottles. Most of this water lies within the cells that make up our muscles, our brain and all the systems of the body. As in their primeval ancestors, these cell masses are immersed in salt water – the tissue fluids – from which they draw nutrients and oxygen, and into which their waste products are excreted. The blood circulation (heart, veins, arteries and capillaries) restores and replenishes this bathing fluid, carrying away the waste products that are excreted in the lungs as carbon dioxide, and by the kidney, mainly as urea. Our source of supplies is the alimentary tract, monitored and controlled by the complex autonomic nervous system, as it feeds and waters the blood on its way to the lungs, where it picks up its vital oxygen supply. The elimination of our waste products by the kidney and bowel means that we lose some of our precious supply of water. Every expired breath contains water vapour, and, throughout the day, the skin loses a little in perspiration. We must make up these losses by consuming 1–2 litres of fresh fluid each day, either from the water we drink or from the liquid elements of our food. Our lives depend on this 'fluid balance'.

If the balance is disturbed, our bodies can become waterlogged or dehydrated and our internal waste products can become poisonous, if allowed to accumulate. As we age, this balancing of intake and output becomes more and more precarious. The autonomic nervous control of intake – as appetite and thirst – can be more easily disturbed. Most acute illnesses create an increased need for fluid, yet it is just in such crises that the appetite and sense of thirst may be depressed in old people. It is common to find an elderly patient refusing more than a spoonful of fluid, when examination reveals a parched tongue, sunken eyes and all the signs of dehydration. Normally the main 'fail-safe' mechanism for such situations lies in the kidney. Increases in concentration or dilution of the blood will be matched by the passage of a small (oliguria) or large (polyuria) flow of urine. However, the aged kidney weakens – it cannot concentrate well so it needs a larger basic volume of water to eliminate the same amount of waste. If, in acute illness, the required water is not being ingested, then the 'fail-safe' mechanism breaks down and the level of urea in the blood begins to rise. Many acutely ill old people show a raised blood urea for this reason. They feel more ill as a result, with further disinclination to drink, and a vicious circle is set up. If this continues for long enough, a complete 'shut down' of kidney function can occur, putting the patient in a desperate situation. Many elderly people are ill for days before they come to the attention of nurses and doctors and therefore have much leeway to make up.

The deficits described above will certainly prolong an old person's disability. Some drugs and medicines can make matters worse too. 'Water tablets' (diuretics), which induce the kidney to discharge salt and water, are excellent for reducing the waterlogging of the tissues (oedema) found especially in heart failure, but they will add insult to injury if the patient is running out of fluids and salt for other reasons. Diabetics are particularly prone to run into these problems when they get ill, and intravenous fluids may be necessary to get them back in balance.

It is evident that a careful watch over the intake and output of fluids is an essential part of sick-bed management of the elderly. 'When in doubt, give fluids' should be the watchword.

BLOOD PRESSURE
Hypertension

'A hundred plus your age' is an old rule of thumb for the systolic blood pressure in adult life. This is now controversial. Long-term studies show that, as blood pressure rises, life expectancy dwindles owing to damage to the brain, heart and blood vessels. Moreover, hypertensives are known to live longer if they are treated. Unfortunately, the elderly have a problem in that the treatment of their hypertension may precipitate a stroke. The emerging solution to this dilemma seems to be that severe elderly hypertension should be treated by a careful selection of the gentlest anti-hypertensive drugs. In such patients, the systolic pressure would usually exceed the 'hundred plus your age' level and the diastolic pressure would be 110 or higher.

Hypotension

Illness tends to lower the blood pressure in old age. The many factors involved in this include fluid balance, the state of the blood vessels and the control exerted by the autonomic nervous system. Some elderly people are particularly liable to suffer a sharp drop of blood pressure in the erect position ('postural' or 'orthostatic' hypotension). Severe attacks will cause fainting and the blood pressure may be temporarily unrecordable. More commonly the patient just feels giddy and his legs may give way. It is important to think of this common condition if an old person keeps pleading to return to bed or if his walking ability shows wide variations at different times of day. A drop of more than 20 mmHg between standing and lying is significant. The most likely cause is a side-effect of medication. This applies especially to the widely used diuretics, and marked postural hypotension calls for their cessation, or, at the very least, a reduction in dose. The condition is often found in convalescence from debilitating illness such as stroke or heart failure. Usually it improves as the patient gains strength. He should be trained slowly to tolerate increasing periods in the upright position. Some intelligent patients learn to calculate how much erect activity they can allow themselves to meet their day-to-day commitments. Where the condition is persistent, elasticated stockings are thought to be helpful. The salt- and water-retaining hormone, fludrocortisone, may be very effective, but fluid balance may be disturbed and the legs may become oedematous. In some cases this is a small price to pay. Anyone who nurses an aged person should ensure that the blood pressure level and its variations are known. If it appears to lie outside the normal range, then it should be monitored daily, like the temperature and pulse.

TEMPERATURE

Except in acute illness, man's internal temperature remains virtually constant throughout life. In old age the homeostatic mechanisms which ensure this may break down, so that over-heating or overcooling is not immediately corrected. In our climate, the latter danger is the prevalent one. Each winter, thousands of old people become hypothermic. Those severely affected seem to lose awareness of how cold they are. They may not think to protect themselves and are sometimes found sitting serenely in an ice-cold room. A common story is of a frail person falling down, when getting out of bed at night to go to the toilet, and, unable to get back to bed, spending the rest of the night on the floor, with only pyjamas or a nightdress for cover. In other cases, hypothermia develops slowly over a number of days, the body's core temperature steadily falling.

Characteristically, hypothermic patients become muddled and confused. Their movements are slow and their limbs stiffen. Their pulse slows, their reflexes are depressed and their blood pressure falls. They feel cold to the touch, not only on the exposed areas but also in areas, such as the lower abdomen, where the skin should be warm. Any temperature below 95°F (35°C) is technically hypothermic but the illness becomes serious below 90°F (32.2°C). Below 85°F (29.8°C) survival is unlikely, although, occasionally, patients have recovered from temperatures much lower than this. There is no immediate remedy apart from slow re-warming – not more than 1°F (0.5°C) is advised. This is achieved by lightly covering the patient in a temperate bedroom and monitoring his temperature carefully. A lightweight aluminium foil space blanket is very effective in preventing further heat loss and in securing a slow recovery. Antibiotics are usually given to counter the broncho-pneumonia which almost inevitably arises. After recovery, rigorous preventive measures, in the form of home heating, home insulation and the provision of appropriate clothing, must be undertaken, because everyone who has suffered from hypothermia is susceptible to it again. In general the clinical thermometer is not a good index of illness in old people. The pulse and respiratory rate are much more sensitive.

PULSE

Rapid pulse (tachycardia)

Healthy old age is not associated with any change in the pulse, although the stiffening of the great vessels makes it easier to feel. The heart rate is, however, much more easily disturbed by exertion, anxiety and illness. A rapid resting pulse (tachycardia) of 100 per minute or more is never normal for old age and an explanation for it must be found (see Table 1).

Table 1 Tachycardia – common causes

Pain	Heart failure
Anxiety	Paroxysmal tachycardia
Infection	Auricular fibrillation
Drugs (e.g., ephedrine)	Pulmonary embolus
Hypoglycaemia	Hyperthyroidism

The likely abnormalities of the heart and lungs are associated also with shortness of breath (dyspnoea). In heart failure associated with tachycardia the pulse chart becomes an excellent measure of improvement in response to therapy, the pulse slowing as the patient recovers. If the old person remains unwell with tachycardia after an infection in the chest, or in some localised area such as an operation wound or leg ulcer, then it may be that the blood has been invaded (septicaemia) – a serious complication. Pulmonary embolus is another possibility. In this condition, clots which have formed in the pelvic or leg veins during the acute illness break off in fragments and are carried in the blood up to, and through, the right side of the heart. Passing into the pulmonary (lung) circulation, they cannot get through the net of capillaries where oxygen and carbon dioxide are exchanged. They stop the flow of blood where they become stuck. Depending on the size and number of these fragments, the effect can range from slight breathlessness, and elevation of the heart rate, to severe heart failure or sudden death. The older one grows, the more likely is this complication, and random autopsy surveys reveal its presence in up to a fifth of cases. It is particularly liable to occur after a fracture of the neck of the femur or after a stroke (the initial clots forming in the affected leg). Treatment is by anticoagulants in suitable cases.

Slow pulse (bradycardia)

This condition is not normal in old age and it may be the vital clue to the cause of the patient's debility (see Table 2).

Table 2 Bradycardia – common causes

Nausea	Coronary thrombosis
Visceral pain	Heart block
Drugs (e.g. digoxin, propranolol)	Sick sinus syndrome
Hypothermia	Carotid sinus syndrome
Hypothyroidism	

Heart-acting drugs, such as digoxin and the beta blockers (e.g. propranolol), should be withdrawn or reduced if the elderly patient develops a markedly slow pulse (say, below 60 per minute). For practical purposes these are the cause until proved otherwise. The slow pulse which may be found in a patient who has recently suffered from a coronary thrombosis is, like nausea and vomiting, usually due to a transient reaction of the autonomic nervous system which governs the heart rate. Sometimes it is the effect of direct cardiac injury which damages the intrinsic pacemaker (the sick sinus syndrome) or its nervous connections with the heart muscle (heart block). Autonomic nerve stimulation cannot then dependably evoke cardiac acceleration when required, and the pulse is usually less than 50 per minute.

Both sick sinus syndrome and heart block often arise without any apparent history of an acute 'coronary'. They can make an old person variably weak and confused, with no other physical signs to explain the symptoms. Electrocardiography makes the diagnosis. The patient's life can be revitalised by the insertion of an artificial pacemaker, and most district general hospitals will undertake this in appropriate cases, irrespective of the patient's age. The procedure is not dangerous and the devices are very reliable.

The carotid sinus syndrome is a curious condition which may

affect the elderly, causing occasional marked slowing of the pulse and fainting attacks (syncope). It arises from an abnormally sensitive reaction of the autonomic nervous system to external pressure on one or other of the large carotid arteries that run up the side of the neck, just at the point where they divide under the angle of the jaw. A tight-fitting collar, or a prescribed cervical collar, can be the cause. On turning the head, the pulse slows and the patient may faint. This is undoubtedly one explanation of the 'queer turns' to which old people are subject, albeit a less common one than postural hypotension.

THE ALIMENTARY TRACT
Nutritional problems

Although taste and smell are said to be somewhat impaired in old age, the elderly generally seem to enjoy their food as much as anyone else. Certainly in institutions the meals constitute the highlight of the day. Food fads can be the result of ill-considered advice (given years before by doctors, nurses or dietitians), which has been so faithfully followed as to become an unbreakable habit. Old age is bound to restrict physical activity, and thus calorie requirements. If appetite is well maintained, then obesity will result, and some invalids will steadily put on weight until they represent a back-breaking nursing problem. A calorie restricted diet then becomes necessary.

Certain dietary deficiencies are common in old people. These include iron (with resultant anaemia) and potassium. Lack of potassium is more likely if diuretics are being taken regularly. It can cause severe, non-specific debility and potassium supplements may be necessary. The two likely vitamin deficiencies are C and D. Widowers who did not learn to prepare proper meals before the death of their wives may not bother to include adequate fruit and vegetables in their diet. They may present with weakness and skin lesions, which prove to be due to scurvy. The B vitamin may be deficient, too – especially in isolates who spend their housekeeping money on alcohol for the comfort it brings. Such deficiencies can aggravate heart failure. Vitamin D is present in barely adequate quantities in the British diet and summer sunshine is needed to supplement this. This supplement is lost by the housebound elderly and Vitamin D is therefore the most widely deficient vitamin in that age group. The resultant weakening of bones (osteomalacia), added to the variable bone thinning (osteoporosis) which all elderly people suffer to some extent, explains, in part, their greater liability to bone fractures. In general, if an old person has been isolated, and is seen to have neglected himself, a daily multivitamin supplement may improve his general condition, irrespective of any other measures that are taken.

Problems of digestion

With the passage of years, one learns to avoid the foods and drink that cause stomach upsets. Armed with this experience, the elderly have few dyspeptic problems, and, when they do occur, they know how to deal with them. The increasingly precarious mechanics of the sphincter between the oesophagus and stomach make older people prone to flatulence (which they take less trouble to contain), but the digestion and absorption of food are generally normal. The liver has vast reserves of function, unless chronically abused by alcohol. However, the internal secretion of insulin by the pancreas is liable to fail, especially in the obese. The majority of diabetics are elderly. The metabolism and elimination of drugs is less certain, and a sizeable proportion of illness in old age is due to this. Often these drugs have been taken in conventional doses and may have caused no trouble to the individual in the past. Any confusional state of recent onset is likely to have been caused by medication and calls for an urgent reappraisal of this. (Chapter 4 deals with drugs and the elderly.)

Bowel function

The main purposes of the large bowel are to store faeces and absorb fluid. Faeces are retained until circumstances are appropriate for their evacuation, during which time fluid is steadily reabsorbed for re-use by the body. The signals of a full rectum are more easily disregarded in old age – especially when physical activity is limited for any reason. Thus, any illness rendering the patient chair-bound or bed-bound will lead to constipation. The longer this continues, the drier and harder the faeces become. They may become so difficult to pass that manual evacuation is necessary. At this stage the abdomen may be distended, and the patient's loss of appetite, along with flatulence and nausea, may resemble the picture of a truly obstructed bowel. Where any of these symptoms are present, rectal examination should be carried out.

Acute illness is doubly likely to produce an impacted rectum because of the associated body fluid depletion that often exists.

Any available water will be absorbed avidly from the increasingly
solid faeces, which thus become even more difficult to pass. A
'ball valve accumulation' may result – a hard rectal mass impossible to extrude, past which liquid faeces slip incontinently.
Prevention is clearly the keynote, the main aims being a regular
toilet routine, an ample fluid intake and minimal full-time bed
rest. The value of bran and roughage is widely acknowledged
although they are not always easy to include in adequate quantities in the sick-room diet of the elderly.

In summing up the sick-room risks run by the elderly, Richard
Asher, a keenly perceptive physician, wrote: 'Look at the patient
lying long in bed. What a pathetic picture he makes! The blood
clotting in his veins, the lime draining from his bones, the scybala
stacking in his colon, the flesh rotting from his seat, the urine
leaking from his distended bladder and the spirit evaporating
from his soul.'

2

COMMON PHYSICAL CONDITIONS OF OLD AGE

DR W. B. WRIGHT

Consultant in Geriatric Medicine,
Querns Hospital, Cirencester

Although our bodily responses to the environment change over the years, everyday diseases and their treatment remain much the same. 'Geriatrics' is really general medicine in this respect. What one wishes to know will be found usually in a good medical textbook. This applies to the management of most infections, nutritional problems, allergic reactions, anaemias and disorders of the endocrine glands. Most injuries receive standard treatment irrespective of age.

Some important conditions become more common, however. This applies particularly to the effects of atheroma (calcifying fatty deposits) in the arteries of the heart, brain and limbs. The resultant strokes, coronary thromboses and limb gangrene cripple a large proportion of the population, but this is not to say that these conditions are primarily due to ageing. Like lung cancer and tobacco smoking, atheromatous arteries may be the long-term effect of some aspect of our way of living. The consumption of too much salt and dairy farm produce is thought to be an important factor. This is taken very seriously in the United States, and it is noteworthy that there has been a sharp decline in cardiovascular disease there in recent years.

Cancer is more common in old people. It would seem that we all have a propensity for developing cancerous change somewhere in the body, given time and aggravating factors, such as tobacco. The skin (rodent ulcer), bowel, breast, lung, prostate gland and stomach are common sites. Adult leukaemia occurs more often in older people. Nevertheless, the importance of this cancer prevalence should not be exaggerated. The sudden removal of all cancer from mankind would have far less effect on chronic invalidism than the elimination of atheroma from the blood vessels.

Infections of the respiratory tract and bladder occur more frequently in the elderly and often complicate other disabling illnesses. It would appear that the defences against infection contained in the blood and tissues of our bodies lose some of their vigour. Virus infections strike harder. Influenza can be a killer in old age. Herpes zoster, or 'shingles', which is due to the chicken-pox virus emerging from a dormant state in the nervous system, can have severe and protracted effects in frail old people. Fungus infections in the mouth, skinfolds and between the toes appear more often. The treatment of these conditions is, of course, essentially the same as in the young.

The elderly seem to grow out of some diseases. Some allergic conditions settle down. Migraine is far less common. Infective hepatitis and acute nephritis are rarely seen. New cases of multiple sclerosis are seldom described, though its apparent disappearance could be due to misdiagnosis.

A few conditions are peculiar to our later years. Some old people are prey to non-specific itching of the skin (senile pruritus) which defies all attempts at diagnosis. 'Pruritus ani' is more common. The benign condition of 'restless legs', which pregnant women suffer, reappears in older people, often tormenting them when they try to get to sleep at night. This is misinterpreted frequently as a restless mind and treated with sedatives. Polymyalgia (temporal arteritis) appears exclusively in old age. Aching of the shoulder and neck muscles occurs and a common feature is headache, a symptom complained of, in general, less often than by the young. If diagnosed correctly (and again there is a great danger of misdiagnosis) it will respond well to treatment with steroids such as prednisone and the patient will make a good recovery.

From a practical management point of view, the diseases relevant to old age can be divided into four groups as follows:

1. Affections of the special senses.
2. Disabling physical conditions.
3. The origins of incontinence.
4. Forms of mental disturbance.

The first three will be dealt with here; the last one will be discussed at length in chapter 3.

AFFECTIONS OF THE SPECIAL SENSES

The two vital special senses, hearing and sight, are those most liable to be damaged by disease, though diabetic neuropathy of the peripheral nerves can impair sensation in the feet so severely that the skin breaks down and chronic indolent ('trophic') ulcers form.

The ears

Some deafness is inevitable, but, in many cases, degenerative changes in the cochlea of the internal ear result in complete hearing loss. The only treatment for this is a hearing aid. Deaf people are now entitled to a free 'behind-the-ear' model, and its maintenance costs. About 25 per cent of elderly ears are loaded with wax, and its removal can improve hearing significantly. Wax will also interfere with the function of a hearing aid and is one of the causes of 'whistling'. The most common cause is a maladjusted volume control. It is a pity that the volume controls cannot be preset and fixed to suit each individual, instead of having to be adjusted each time the aid is switched on, because old people have great difficulty in fiddling with the controls. This, and the resultant whistling of maladjustment, cause many to give up trying to use the aid. These problems are so widespread that voluntary organisations have been set up in many areas, specifically to instruct and encourage those who have recently been prescribed a hearing aid.

Some elderly people prefer to use the old-fashioned horn in their own homes, as the quality of the sound is better. Various 'communicators' are available. They are held by a companion or nurse and can be amplified to a greater extent than the personal aid. Deaf people can hear best when they do not have to cope with a medley of sounds. If the radio is playing, it is better to switch it off than shout over the background noise. Shouting and other loud noises can make things worse because of a phenomenon called 'recruitment' which so distorts the sound in the inner ear as to make it seem very excessive.

Deafness develops very slowly, and ways of overcoming the disability can be learned. Some deaf old people are good lip-readers, therefore it is important to face the patient squarely, to ensure that your lips can be seen.

Tinnitus

Described as ringing, singing or buzzing in the ears, tinnitus is experienced by up to 15 per cent of the elderly. It is caused usually by degenerative changes in the inner ear, though it is a known side-effect of overdosage with aspirin, quinine and occasional other drugs. It is associated to some degree with deafness, and impacted ear wax is a likely aggravating factor, both symptoms improving when this is cleared. A good hearing aid can help, since the better audibility of external sounds diverts attention away from the tinnitus.

Menière's disease is a distressing composite of severe giddiness, deafness and tinnitus, coming in clusters of attacks, and is due to abnormal pressure changes in the internal ear. Symptomatic treatment with various medicines will help initially, but the condition is often progressive, ending in absolute deafness. Where the symptoms are extreme, it may be necessary to anticipate this by ending inner ear function artificially.

The eyes

Conjunctivitis is a common, recurrent problem for old people. Old eyelids are less resilient in following the contours of the eyeball and the space between traps infection more easily, thus a red eye is often seen. The trouble usually responds promptly to antibiotic eye ointment. It is worth taking a more careful look at the eyelids when conjunctivitis persistently recurs, because entropion may be present. This means that the lower eyelid has flipped inwards so that the eyelashes sweep the eyeball. Old people's eyelid lashes are so sparse that it can be difficult to be sure of this. Pull the skin of the lower lid down gently and the lashes will suddenly appear. A small incision and suture below the lower lid will put this right.

Certain conditions can cause visual failure, as follows:

Hardening of the eye lens

This accounts for the long-sightedness of advancing age, and it must be remembered that this is a continuous process and that corrective spectacles must be changed regularly.

Cataract

Cataracts are caused by an accumulation of opacities in the lens which interfere with vision. Much more likely in diabetics, this common form of visual damage impairs central vision first, so that the patient can 'see around it' to some extent. Bright light makes things worse, for the lens opacities 'flare' like fog particles in headlamps, so dark glasses help at an early stage. When visual impairment reaches a certain level, and if the eye is otherwise healthy, the lens should be removed. Thick 'pebble lens' glasses have to be worn as these heavy lenses are necessary to replace the extracted original. Nowadays an acrylic replacement can be inserted into the eye, or soft contact lenses can be worn.

Glaucoma

The eye is essentially a tense bag of fluid which is constantly in balance between drainage and replacement. This balance can be disturbed by severe fluid depletion and it is for this reason that some old people notice a change in their eyesight during or after illness. Much more serious is an obstructed drainage system. Glaucoma, which is the result, can permanently damage or destroy the sight of the affected eye. Acute glaucoma is an agonizingly painful loss of vision which may quickly make the old person ill and delirious. The eye becomes inflamed; the pupil looks cloudy and loses its perfectly circular shape. These signs call for immediate specialist intervention or the eye will lose its sight irrevocably.

Chronic glaucoma is an insidious, slow-developing disease, and there may be no complaint of pain. The patient's vision dims and sometimes haloes may be seen around lights. 'Tunnel' vision may occur (the peripheral visual fields being obscured), and measurement reveals an increased tension of the eye. In mild cases the condition can be controlled by eye drops which open the drainage channels more widely; otherwise surgical intervention will be required.

Retinal damage

The highly specialised retinal cells and their nervous connections are extremely vulnerable to any disease that affects their small nutrient vessels. The inflammatory lesions of temporal arteritis will cause blindness if the disease is not diagnosed and treated expeditely. Far more common is the vascular damage of hypertension and diabetes, and the treatment of these is much more difficult. Regular retinal examination of such patients is mandatory. New techniques, such as the use of lasers, can halt visual deterioration, for a time at least. Unfortunately, much retinal degeneration, including the 'senile macular' type which affects central vision, is irreversible.

In the presence of severe visual impairment, one must turn to visual aids – the magnifying viewer, large-print reading books, and the like. Blind registration can bring a variety of benefits and should be pursued.

DISABLING PHYSICAL CONDITIONS

Though old age brings frailty, it should not of itself be regarded as disabling. Doctors and nurses who leave disability undiagnosed, except as 'ageing', do a great disservice to the patient and his attendants. Certainly some of the likely diseases are irreversible, but others are not, and these can be distinguished. A good rule of thumb which will introduce more objectivity into one's thinking when observing an old person who has great difficulty in getting about, is to ask: 'Is this difficulty due to *weakness, stiffness* or *pain?*' (see Table 3).

Table 3 Definitions of disability

Weakness	Stiffness	Pain
Debility (cardiac, toxic, metabolic, etc.)	Ankylosis	Osteoarthritis
	Arthrodesis	Rheumatoid arthritis
Disinclination (depression)	Parkinsonism	Gout
	Spasticity	Polymyalgia
Disuse (confinement to bed, chair)		Paget's disease
		Injury
Paresis (stroke, cervical spondylosis, etc.)		Painful foot conditions

The definition of a problem is the first step towards its solution. To decide into which of these broad categories the patient's problem falls is a major step towards effective action in some cases. Old people's symptoms are often muted and sometimes misleading. Weakness or pain may be misinterpreted as stiffness, and vice versa. A limping old man may have to be asked: 'Are you in pain when you walk?' before admitting that this is, indeed, the case. Generalised 'rheumatism' may be the complaint when closer observation reveals that only one joint, such as an injured or inflamed hip, is involved significantly. If the inflammation of that joint is severe, acute and associated with a marked general deterioration, then the 'arthritis' could be the not uncommon example of a joint infection picked up from the blood. Any sudden increase in disability calls for an adequate explanation. An old man, complaining of aches and pains, may not mention that he fell the day before and that the problem lies in the rib cage, where one or more fractures may exist.

'Joint pains' can be pains in the muscles (e.g. bruising or polymyalgia) or the bones (e.g. tumour deposits or Paget's disease). An old person with a fractured femur may never walk again if the hip girdle weakness which caused the fall is overlooked, and the Vitamin D deficiency which caused this, and the bone brittleness, is never corrected. A slightly hemiplegic limb may become irreversibly spastic because of unrelieved osteoarthritic pain in the hip or knee of that side. The arthritis which restricts all activity may really be trivial in comparison with the obesity and heart failure that are the real culprits. Attendants who overemphasise the disabling role of old age will fall into all these traps, unnecessarily consigning many of their elders to a permanent invalid life.

The nervous system

Stroke

A stroke is caused by clotting or bleeding of the brain's nutrient vessels. Almost any part can be compromised in this way, but the middle cerebral area is usually affected with resultant paralysis of the face, arm and leg on the opposite side. Haemorrhage has a more dramatic onset and carries a worse outlook than thrombosis. It often occurs during vigorous activity or emotional upset. Headache may be severe and drowsiness or stupor is likely. Thrombosis is not associated with headache and usually occurs on waking in the morning, or after a daytime nap. Needless to say, the older the patient, the deeper any initial stupor, and the more severe the paralysis, the worse is the outlook. Stroke damage is usually maximal at onset, with slow recovery beginning within a week or two and tailing off over many months. Paralysis can be complete, or so slight as to escape notice at first.

In the early days, the full extent of the damage must be appraised. Certain specific points must be checked as follows:

1. Is there a flicker of movement anywhere in the affected arm or leg? Early finger movement should mean good arm recovery; any ankle movement should mean that walking will be possible.
2. Is sensation affected? Failure to appreciate touch or pin-

prick, a tendency to ignore the paralysed side, or failure to identify the affected limb, all mean that the damage has extended from the motor into the sensory cerebral cortex.

3. Is balance preserved? Can the patient sit up without falling to one side? This is one of the things which recovers earliest, and the patient's independence hangs on it.

4. Can the patient see objects in the field of vision (i.e. 'out of the corner of his eye') on the paralysed side? If not, the optic tracts leading to the visual centre of the brain have been interrupted.

5. Is speech damaged? A stroke can make the pronunciation of words slurred and difficult (dysarthria), but, more seriously, it can damage the speech centre so that the brain cannot think of the necessary words to convey meaning (dysphasia).

6. Quite apart from any speech defect, is the patient's thinking confused? Anything more than trivial mental disturbance makes it impossible to retrain the patient towards independence. What has been taught will have been forgotten by the next morning.

A methodical appraisal of these six points will give a much greater understanding of the patient's disability and his chances.

The psychological effect of a stroke on the patient and his family is very considerable, and efficient nursing must always take this into account. The family and the patient must be trained jointly to manage the disability. Relatives must be given targets and responsibilities so that they come to see the patient as halfway to recovery, rather than half dead. Towards this end, rehabilitation must be carried out at home, at least part of the time. The patient should succeed in his efforts, so each step towards independence must be small enough to be successful. If, in spite of this, he cannot be jogged out of despair, antidepressant therapy is sometimes helpful.

Complications specific to stroke include spasm (spasticity) of the affected arm and leg, and dislocation downwards (subluxation) of the paralysed shoulder. Good management, in co-operation with the physiotherapist, can avert these. Heel sores on the weak side are so likely that a foot cradle for all stroke patients is a wise precaution.

Cervical spondylosis

Degenerative changes in the bones and spinal joints affect the neck, at least to some extent, universally. In some cases neck flexion becomes so severe that a supporting collar has to be fitted. The combination of osteoarthritis of the spinal joints and neck flexion can interfere with the blood supply to the spinal cord, lying in its bony tunnel. Varying degrees of paralysis of both arms and legs can result. The affected legs behave in exactly the same way as if stroke damage had occurred, with the same spastic tendency, but the patient's brain function is normal in all respects. The supportive collar and physiotherapy can help what is otherwise a progressive condition.

Parkinson's disease

When an amateur actor tries to imitate a very old person, he flexes his head, his back and his arms, his hands tremble, he adopts a monotonous voice, and shuffles across the stage with little steps. This is not old age. It is Parkinson's disease as it affects the elderly. Parkinson's disease results from degeneration of what is called the extra-pyramidal nervous system, a collection of nerve centres and tracts at the base of the brain, and in the spinal cord, which is responsible for smoothing out willed movements within a background of good body posture. The disease usually begins in middle life and extends into old age. It is nearly always missed in the early stages, being accepted as the natural changes of age. The stiffening and weakening of body musculature will make any other disability, such as arthritis, or mild stroke damage, that much more likely to defeat the patient, and tip the scales towards chronic invalidism.

A useful early sign of Parkinson's disease is a change in handwriting, which becomes smaller (micrographia) and shakier. (The disease has occasionally been diagnosed by letter!) There is now effective treatment. It has been found that there is a deficiency of a substance called dopamine in the Parkinsonian brain. Its replacement strikingly improves the weakness and rigidity of the body muscles. Dopamine cannot be taken by mouth but a related substance, L-dopa, can. Given with a supportive enzyme in a combined tablet, L-dopa quickly restores better movement in up to three-quarters of Parkinsonian patients. There are side-effects and long-term problems. The drug is especially likely to cause mental disturbance in mildly confused subjects. Intensive research is currently being carried out in order to find answers to the difficulties that have arisen in the use of what is, at times, a spectacularly successful therapy.

This research could help to improve the function of the brain in senile dementia.

Joint diseases

'Creaking hinges hang the longest' runs the saying. This shows an awareness that the common joint problems of old age aren't much more than a nuisance. Most gnarled old fingers are osteoarthritic, but they are seldom more than occasionally stiff and painful. Aching joints in the neck and back, particularly marked the day after unaccustomed exercise, have the same origins, and the milder cases respond well to various forms of local heat, gentle exercise and analgesic tablets. Osteoarthritis of the hip is a disabling condition that is now amenable to treatment. The condition may be quite asymmetrical, being far more severe on one side than the other. Any old joint injury seems to attract osteoarthritic change, as does habitual bad posture. Characteristically, the joint cartilage wears away, baring the bone ends to each other. There is some surrounding inflammation and swelling. Spicules of new bone form around the joint (exostoses). The joint may finally become fixed and immobile (ankylosis). Usually the leg shortens. It tends to rotate externally, so that the knee bends sideways and a 'scissoring gait' develops. Sitting and standing become mechanically difficult, and the patient is severely encumbered.

Nowadays, such cases are candidates for total surgical replacement of the hip. This operation can be considered almost irrespective of age, provided that the subject is in otherwise reasonable health. The whole head of the femur is removed and replaced by a metal prosthesis, fitted into a cup of strong acrylic material, that is fixed to the pelvis. A successful hip replacement will restore near normal joint function and will last an elderly person for the rest of his life. If necessary, both sides can be dealt with.

The knee may suffer as badly as the hip; its lateral ligaments may be so damaged that the lower leg begins to splay sideways, giving a severe 'knock-knee' effect. Operations have been devised to restore knee function, but they are not yet as successful as those for the hip. Sometimes the knee has to be arthrodesed (fixed rigidly) in the extended position to enable the patient to continue some walking at least.

Fractured femur

It is appropriate to mention this condition because, in spite of surgical intervention, a great deal of invalidism still results from this fracture. An important reason for this is the likelihood that those who fall so heavily as to break the femur may well have been suffering latent debility at the time, which is then compounded by the fracture. Examples commonly discovered are mild stroke damage, dementing states, myxoedema, malnutrition, osteomalacia and arthritis. Recovery is therefore slow and incomplete. Such patients' post-operative progress can be interrupted by a variety of complications (see Table 4).

Table 4 Complications after fracture of the femur

Bronchopneumonia	Pressure sore (heel)
Fluid balance upset	Deep venous thrombosis
Poor mental state after anaesthesia	Fat embolism

If an old person's progress after surgery is poor, it is wise to assume that some other condition, apart from the injury and operation, has been present or is developing; put cryptically: Operation + X = disability. Find X.

The heart and circulation

'You are as old as your arteries'. There is some evidence that modification of our diet and way of life may mitigate the harshness of this truth, but the truth must be faced that chronic obstruction of the blood vessels to the heart, brain and limbs is the predominating disabler. The coronary arteries are a prime example. From early middle age onwards, accumulating atheroma in these vital nutrient vessels to the heart muscle leave them a prey to clot formation, with catastrophic results. The sudden death of middle-aged men is nearly always due to this. Failing blood supply through these constricted vessels is the origin of the crushing chest pain on exercise known as angina pectoris. As age advances, coronary artery disease continues inexorably, yet the picture of heart disease is much less dramatic. Angina becomes less and less common, but cardiac insufficiency and failure more and more prevalent. It may be that the aged cannot walk or exercise vigorously enough to bring out the anginal pain, or the sensory nerves may no longer register it.

Where the coronary arteries are badly affected, cardiac reserves dwindle so that less and less exercise can be tolerated without exhaustion and breathlessness. The cardiac output falls and those who formerly were hypertensive may appear to reassume a normal blood pressure, which is in fact below their requirements.

Heart failure

This is the result of coronary artery disease or hypertension in most cases, although multiple clots in the lungs, arising from thrombosis in the deep veins of the legs or pelvis, are a common cause. Occasionally, chronic bronchitis or other obstructive diseases of the lung airways may be responsible, but respiratory cripples tend to die before they reach old age.

The classic signs are breathlessness, which may make it impossible for the patient to lie down (orthopnoea), distended veins (seen most easily in the neck), and the accumulation of fluid in the legs, trunk and lungs (oedema). Except in specific instances (e.g. heart block), the pulse is rapid. The patient usually looks ill and sometimes slightly blue (cyanosis). Mild heart failure can complicate any other problem sufficiently to disable the patient. Note must be taken of any undue breathlessness on slight effort, or of fatigue too easily induced. These may indicate that heart failure is developing. Nowadays, drugs which produce an increased drainage of body water and salt through the kidneys (diuretics or 'water tablets') are the mainstay of treatment. They rapidly reduce the congestion of the lungs, and throughout the body, enabling the patient to recover his breath and energy. An intravenous diuretic injection can be life-saving. Digitalis, the foxglove extract (digoxin), is used much less than formerly for its direct restorative effect on cardiac muscle and heart rate.

Very occasionally, heart failure is cured by treating an overactive thyroid gland (thyrotoxicosis) which has overloaded the heart beyond its reserves. This must be thought of particularly when the heart rate remains rapid and completely irregular (auricular fibrillation), in spite of conventional treatment, or if there is a previous, or family, history of thyroid trouble. Elderly heart failure responds quite well to treatment as a rule and it should be possible to get the patient back in balance, but its development undoubtedly carries significance as regards shortened life expectancy.

Ischaemia of limbs

Restricted blood supply to the limbs is usually associated with cardiovascular disease elsewhere, so that the patient may have a history of heart disease or stroke damage. Sometimes the blood supply to a limb is abruptly obstructed by a clot which has formed in the heart or on an atheromatous patch in one of the great arteries, such as the aorta. The effect is similar to the application of a tourniquet. The pulses of the limb below the clot disappear and the skin becomes cold and pale, with a bluish tint. Unless, as sometimes happens in diabetics, the sensory nerves of the limb have been damaged, limb pain is increasingly severe. Surgery is urgently needed if there is to be any hope of extracting the clot in time to save the limb, otherwise the ischaemic area will die (gangrene) and, unless it is very localised, will have to be removed by amputation. The use of vascular grafts has made corrective surgery much more successful than it used to be, so every patient in this stricture should have the benefit of a surgical opinion.

The circulation to the legs is more often chronically obstructed. This does not have the dramatic effects described in the previous paragraph. Intermittent claudication may be the first symptom. Characteristically, the sufferer can walk symptomlessly for a certain distance. A dull pain then grips the calf muscles, stopping him. He goes on again, only to be stopped after a similar distance. Limbs with a poor blood supply may become deathly pale when elevated. When they are lowered a beetroot red colour may develop (Buerger's sign). Scaling may appear around the ankles, and the nails may deteriorate. Any slight injury is liable to cause an ulcer, which will be very slow to heal. This is particularly true in diabetes. If the obstruction to the circulation is localised to one or two sites in the larger blood vessels, reconstructive surgery can be carried out with excellent results. It seems likely also that certain medication, taken routinely, may prevent recurrences.

Leg ulcers

Ulceration of the legs usually results from disruption within the network of leg veins, due either to chronic untreated varicosities or to a long-term effect of previous deep venous thrombosis in the calf. In either case, the little venous valves stationed at intervals along the main channels break down and can no longer hold the weight of the erect leg's long column of blood. The tissues around the ankle are most vulnerable to the resultant venous back pressure, becoming boggy with oedema and starved of fresh blood. Over a period of time the overlying skin may become oozy, eczematous and pigmented. With much oedema, small flabby blisters will erupt, forming itchy scales as they dry. The leg will ulcerate readily over a rapidly widening area in response to any injury. Scratching is a common cause of injury and is a major cause of ulceration. It can go on for months or years, and should be suspected, even when the patient is unaware of doing it.

The treatment of ulcers has been the object of fads and fancies over many years, but certain good rules emerge as follow:

1. Get the oedema out of the area. If the patient puts on well-fitting elasticated stockings on rising each morning, oedematous swelling can be kept away from the ulcerated area. These stockings are uncomfortable and unpopular. An elastic bandage usually works better, but can't easily be applied personally by the patient. Diuretics (water tablets) sometimes help, but less than might be expected, because it is an obstructive, rather than generalised, oedema that is being treated. Raising the foot of the bed, so that the affected leg is elevated all night, is an excellent measure, always worthy of adoption. Propping up the leg on a stool is less valuable as care must be taken not to support the leg's whole weight solely on the heel, which could well break down and ulcerate. Resting on top of the covers of a bed which has been raised at the bottom is much safer. Indeed, a period of this kind of bed rest is the fastest way to get control of a deteriorating ulcer.

2. Protect the area from further damage. Very frequent dressings which stick to the raw area are sure to hurt the patient and his delicate new forming tissues. A very popular and successful dressing nowadays is a zinc paste bandage, which can be wound on and off easily, and may remain in place for a week. An elasticated bandage may be applied on top. One great advantage is that the patient can't get his hands on it!

3. Antibiotics should be given systemically, rather than locally, if they are needed. Local reactions to antibiotics and, indeed, many other substances applied to raw ulcers are common. As far as applications are concerned, the blander they are the better.

THE ORIGINS OF INCONTINENCE

Everybody is incontinent at some time in life, if only in child-hood. The occasional 'dribble' can occur during moments of stress, mental or physical, in any adult. This usually amounts to transient loss of control owing to an over-full bladder, combined with sudden exertion, fright or laughter. Obviously the elderly run a bigger risk of such accidents, but, as a general rule, healthy old people are no more incontinent than anybody else. Persistent incontinence in old age should be therefore investigated, and treated as an abnormality, rather than be dismissed as inevitable.

Any acute illness can precipitate incontinence. The original problem could be anything from a virus infection to a stroke. About half of those patients admitted to the average geriatric unit are incontinent on arrival. In most cases this clears up as the illness resolves. Any degree of dementia makes the patient far more vulnerable to this complication, which is then more likely to be persistent. The longer any incontinence persists, the more difficult it is to reverse. Habitual incontinence is one of the most common causes of rejection by the supporting family.

A hunt for pelvic abnormalities is often disappointing but cystitis (bladder infection) is commonly present and must be treated. Any acute illness may be associated with the develop-ment of impacted constipation in the rectum. Clearing this could also relieve the incontinence. Rectal examination is therefore essential where this is likely. At the same time, such aggravating factors as intertrigo or thrush, and inflammation in the vagina or urethra, should be sought. An excessive flow of urine (poly-uria) can be the cause. One particular example of this is un-treated diabetes. The urine should therefore be tested for sugar. Polyuria can also be caused by diuretics (water tablets), and, in some institutions, the cutting down of such medication has resulted in a considerable improvement in the incidence of the problem.

Anything that makes an old person less likely to heed the call to the toilet can provoke incontinence. Sedatives, tranquillizers and sleeping tablets are all culpable in this respect and should be stopped, or at least cut down, if possible. The very fact of lying in bed impairs initiative. Many elderly patients regain control of their bladder as soon as they are well enough to sit in a chair. This is one of the reasons for the advocated early ambulation of the elderly sick. The first step in general management should be to ensure easy toilet access; a commode should be placed beside the bed, if necessary.

Any initial distress that is felt by the incontinent patient quickly passes as the episodes recur, and he or she may have to be trained out of the habit. Regular toileting, with carefully recorded observations of the pattern of the incontinence, is successful more often than might be expected. Frequently it becomes possible to anticipate the incontinence and so prevent it. The interest of all concerned, including the patient, quickens as improvement is observed.

In many elderly patients, slight degenerative changes in the nervous system between the brain and the bladder make the normal control of emptying signals much less easy. One way to deal with this is to reduce the 'irritability' of the bladder – that is, to damp down its impulses to contract. There are several drugs on the market designed to do this. Emepronium and flavoxate hydrochloride are two examples. Their effect is variable and not always successful; indeed, in some cases they may appear to worsen the condition. If so, chronic retention of urine with 'overflow' incontinence is a possibility. The usefulness of other groups of drugs, including the 'anti-prostaglandins' and the 'calcium antagonists', is being investigated at present. At some hospitals, urodynamic studies of bladder function reveal types of incontinence that respond to specific treatment with drugs or other measures. Often, attendance at a day hospital is associated with a prompt improvement, probably for psychological reasons analogous to those operating when a child first begins to attend school.

When none of these measures has been successful, and the incontinence is beyond control with the various pads and pants available, condom-type drainage for men or indwelling catheterisation for women may have to be instituted. These devices can now drain into catheter bags concealed under the clothing so that they are not visible. It is important to do this early enough to ensure that family goodwill has not run out. With catheterisation urinary infection always results, but, in most cases, this infection neither invades nor troubles the patient. Sometimes the catheter can be removed after several weeks without a recurrence of incontinence, provided that the patient's vitality has improved sufficiently. If the 'catheter option' is borne in mind, most elderly invalids can be kept dry at home.

Further information

An increasing number of nurses are working as Continence Advisers, attached to District Health Authorities, giving help and advice to incontinent patients and to those caring for them. The Association of Continence Advisers has produced a comprehensive catalogue of incontinence aids and equipment of all kinds, which may be obtained from The Secretary, Association of Continence Advisers, c/o The Disabled Living Foundation, 346 Kensington High Street, London W14 8NS. The Disabled Living Foundation also has an Incontinence Adviser who will give up-to-date information and advice about aids and equipment and the general management of incontinence.

Further reading

Mandelstam, Dorothy (Ed.), *Incontinence and its Management* (Croom Helm Ltd, London).

3
PSYCHIATRIC DISORDERS IN THE ELDERLY

DR JOHN WATTIS

Consultant in the Psychiatry of Old Age,
St James's Hospital, Leeds

The possibility of mental illness is one of the most frightening aspects of old age. Many old people are terrified of 'going senile' and it is only in the last 25 years or so that doctors have realised that there are many different forms of mental illness in old age, some of which can be cured, and in some of which the suffering of the patient and his relatives can at least be alleviated. Some old people, remembering the workhouses and asylums, fear that any signs of mental illness will result in incarceration. This 'removals and storage' concept of the psychiatric medicine of old age has now been replaced by an approach based on the careful assessment of the patient in his or her own environment, and the judicious use of community support services and short-term hospital admission, so that, in most cases, admission to a long-stay mental hospital, or even to an old people's home, is avoided.

Mental illness is not easy to define. What can be said is that, when a person's behaviour is seriously out of step with his surroundings, the label of 'mental illness' is likely to be applied. This discrepancy between the behaviour of the person and his environment can, however, result from causes other than mental illness. Even when mental illness is undoubtedly present, other factors may be responsible for worsening the situation to the point where outside intervention is called for.

Figure 1 shows how various factors interact to produce behaviour which we label 'mental illness'. The old person's surroundings are perceived through the special senses, especially sight and hearing, and the brain then processes this

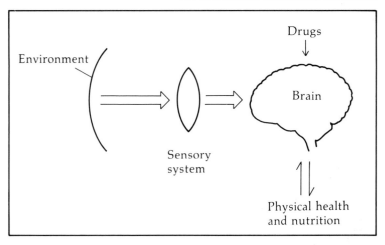

Fig. 1 Interactive model of mental illness in old age.

information and initiates appropriate behaviour. The processing ability of the brain may be limited by intrinsic disorders, some of which are the result of damage to the structure of the brain and some of which are probably due to biochemical malfunctions. The way the person copes with changes in the outside world will be affected also by the ways in which he or she has learned to cope with changes in the past. These ways of coping ('strategies') may never have been very appropriate and may be inadequate to the task of coping with the stresses of old age. For example, a man may have taken refuge from the difficulties of family life by putting all his energy into his work. He then retires and is thrown into close contact with his wife. She has no space for him in the household routine, and he, feeling useless, becomes morose and depressed.

The functioning of the brain can be affected by physical ill health or nutrition and by medication (drugs) prescribed for physical and psychiatric illnesses.

An old lady, who lived alone, had a poor memory and tended to get muddled, but coped with the help of a neighbour and social services. One day she turned the home help away, claiming that the house did not belong to her so that she had no authority to allow the home help in. She was also, at this time, found to be neglecting herself and not eating. Medical examination showed that the patient had pneumonia. The extra stress that physical ill health had produced increased confusion and made the patient unable to cope.

The importance of the model summarised in Fig. 1 is that it emphasises how problems in more than one area may interact to produce a cumulative effect on behaviour. A step-by-step analysis of problems can be made, and this chapter is set out to facilitate that kind of analysis.

ENVIRONMENT

If the circumstances in which people live, either at home or at work, are sufficiently stressful, they will begin eventually to behave in an abnormal fashion. We have probably all caught ourselves losing our temper with our children, or other people, when we have been feeling overtired or have had a headache. Soldiers exposed to extreme stress in wartime conditions, or hostages in terrorist attacks, may suffer psychological damage, and this has recently been the topic of discussion in the newspapers. As a matter of course, old people have to cope with many stresses. They are usually in the situation of compulsory unemployment and there may be resultant poverty and loss of status. In addition, many of their old friends and relatives may have died and the old person has to cope with the sorrow of these bereavements. Physical health may be waning, too, sometimes with consequent decline in activity and social contact. In these circumstances, it is surprising that more old people do not suffer from psychological disturbances.

Managing change

Partly because of poor eyesight and hearing, and partly, in some cases, because of a decline in mental agility, many old people find it difficult to cope with sudden change. An old person who develops a physical illness and is rushed off to hospital may become confused simply because of the changes to which he is subject. Whenever an old person does have to move from familiar surroundings into hospital or an old people's home, the change must be managed carefully. This is especially important if the old person is confused for other reasons. Time should be taken to explain, repeatedly, if necessary, what is happening, and why. Whenever possible, transition from one environment to another should be gradual, but even an emergency admission to hospital can be managed successfully if ambulancemen, nursing staff and others take time to appreciate the patient's position, and explain to him what is going on. The presence of a relative, or other known and trusted person, throughout the transitional period is of great benefit, as the old person has someone to whom he can relate whilst the necessary changes are taking place.

Supportive environment

If somebody loses a leg, an artificial limb is provided. Similarly, the simple expedient of keeping a list of things to do may prove helpful for someone whose memory is failing. Even elderly people with poor memories, living alone, can be helped by careful planning of quite simple measures. For example, a telephone call in the morning may remind the person what day of the week it is and that she has to get up and get dressed. Institutional environments, such as hospitals and old people's homes, can be designed to provide the maximum information for those with poor memories. Toilets should be clearly marked with signs that can be read at a distance, and colour coding of toilet doors may prove helpful for the confused patient. On a psychiatric ward for old people, the patient's first name should be written in large letters on a label attached to the wardrobe adjacent to his bed. Architects designing environments for old people need to imagine themselves in the situation where their eyesight is not very good and where they may be a little perplexed, and then plan the surroundings so that as many clues as possible are given to help confused old people to orientate themselves. One old people's home I visited (a converted old house) had such a complicated floor plan that I became lost as I was led around. In addition, although the toilet doors had been thoughtfully colour-coded, unfortunately, the same colour scheme had been used for the kitchen doors!

Special techniques

In addition to careful design, or modification of the environment, a thoughtful approach by relatives and staff can alleviate the problems of confused patients. 'Reality orientation' is the name given to a technique intended to improve the confused patient's contact with the outside world. Helpers are taught to approach patients as individuals, providing them with appropriate information to increase contact with reality, and involving them in making decisions. For example, instead of simply telling the patient to 'get up' in the morning, the nurse will approach the patient, call him by name, and explain that he is in hospital, thus providing reassurance. She will identify herself as a nurse and will say that breakfast will be ready in half an hour, in order that he has time to get up. In addition to this 'background reality orientation', some units provide specific group or individual activities designed to improve the patient's contact with important aspects of reality. These take the form of 'classroom' sessions in which patients are encouraged to pay attention to the weather and the place they are in, and to recognise common objects. They may be encouraged also to use a calendar and clock to keep in touch with time, and to discuss recent happenings.

Another technique, which, paradoxically, often helps to improve an old person's contact with reality, is reminiscence. Here, on an individual basis or in a group, the patient is encouraged to talk about his past life. Old pictures of the area in which he lived, tape recordings and occupational items can all be used to stimulate memories. For some confused patients, talking about the past is relatively easy and, once they begin to talk and take an interest, conversation can be directed into areas more relevant to everyday life. For the depressed patient, too, reminiscence can be used to increase self-esteem and combat depressive feelings of unworthiness.

Bereavement

In western society, bereavement is uncommon in younger age groups and death is usually associated with old age. Most old people cope well with bereavement, especially if supported by someone willing to listen. Nevertheless, loss of the spouse for someone who has been married, perhaps for 40 or 50 years, can be shattering. After bereavement a short period of numbness is followed usually by grief and sometimes a certain amount of withdrawal from other relationships. Even in normal grief, people sometimes imagine that they can hear the voice of their loved one, and may feel compelled to visit places which hold memories of the dead person. A degree of lack of concentration and disorganisation is quite normal also. Most people find it helpful to have a friend or relative who will allow them to talk about their feelings for the dead person and reassure them that their tears and feeling of depression are normal.

Sometimes grief may be prolonged unduly and skilled help may be necessary to help the bereaved person talk about his feelings. The most common feeling is guilt over some difficulties in the relationship with the deceased person, and the bereaved may need a good deal of help to talk about these feelings openly, in order that grieving is completed. Bereavement may also precipitate a depressive illness needing treatment in its own right. It can sometimes unmask dementia too. Whilst alive, the spouse may have compensated for increasing memory difficulties in the bereaved person, but, following the death of the spouse, these memory defects may be exposed and the demented old person may suddenly become unable to cope.

SENSES

In some 'brain washing' techniques, prisoners are blindfolded and kept in silence to produce confusion and to render them more amenable to interrogation. This is called sensory deprivation. Few healthy young people appreciate the degree of relative sensory deprivation suffered by some old people. Hearing impairment may put the old person out of contact with reality and others may mistakenly see this as evidence of 'confusion'.

> Two elderly sisters lived with an elderly friend. One of the sisters, suffering from dementia, became quite confused and her behaviour became bizarre. The friend suspected that the second sister was suffering from dementia, too. On interview, however, it became apparent that the second sister was not hearing most of the questions addressed to her, and, when she was provided with a temporary hearing aid, all signs of 'confusion' disappeared. She has since been fitted with a permanent hearing aid and her friend now complains that she has to be careful what she says!

Some old people develop persecutory ideas, believing that others are talking behind their backs or even plotting against them. Deafness is unusually common in this group and may contribute to the development of the condition. Poor eyesight can isolate an old person, too. There may be lack of confidence in going out of the house and difficulty in reading, leading to loss of contact with current affairs. Sometimes, all that is required is an appropriate pair of spectacles. In other cases, cataracts may be developing which require operation. In yet other cases, there may be no way to save the person's sight. The patient should then be registered as partially sighted or blind, through his doctor. Social service departments and voluntary groups run special clubs, and may provide 'talking books' and other aids for sight-impaired people, all of which can be made available once the person is 'registered'.

PSYCHIATRIC ILLNESSES

Traditionally, these disorders are divided into neuroses and psychoses. One American psychiatrist joked that neurotics build castles in the air, psychotics live in them and psychiatrists collect the rent. This encapsulates the main difference between neuroses and psychoses, in that the latter involve loss of contact with reality. Neurotic disorders are probably best regarded as a result of the patient learning unsatisfactory ways of coping ('strategies') with the stresses and strains of life, and their roots often go back to earlier life experiences. An inherited tendency to be anxious may contribute to the development of these conditions. For example, a child may be afraid of going to school. She may become sufficiently anxious to refuse to go. A mother who is anxious herself may openly, or inadvertently, encourage this behaviour. When the girl grows up, she will have learned to deal with anxiety-provoking situations by avoiding them. If she has a successful marriage, she may be sufficiently secure not to develop any problems. Then, perhaps in old age, her husband becomes ill and her anxiety level increases. She becomes afraid to leave the house without her husband's company and cannot go into crowded places at all. This makes her even more anxious and sets up a vicious circle which eventually incapacitates her to the extent that psychiatric help is sought. That help will probably take the form of first excluding physical illness that can produce a similar picture and then, possibly with the help of a psychologist, exploring the patient's problems and teaching her to relax, in order that she can gradually relearn her ability to cope with stressful situations.

Psychotic disorders, as well as involving loss of contact with reality, tend to be more severe. They can be subdivided into the organic disorders which involve structural changes in the brain and the functional disorders which are presumed to be due to biochemical malfunction. Acute confusional states, owing to the effects of physical illness on the brain, are usually classified as a subdivision of organic disorders, but are dealt with separately in this chapter under the heading of physical health and nutrition. Figure 2 summarises a simple classification of mental disorders.

Organic structural disorders

Senile dementia of the Alzheimer type (SDAT) is the most common organic disorder in old age. Alzheimer was the pathol-

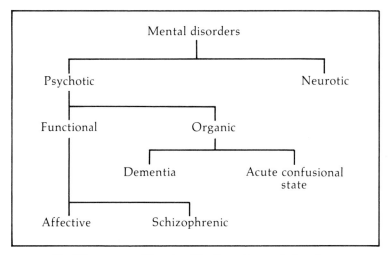

Fig. 2 Summary of the classification of mental disorders.

ogist who identified the microscopic structural changes in the brain associated with this disease. The brain of a person suffering from this disorder is often shrunken, and numerous microscopic areas of damage called 'senile plaques' can be identified. These disrupt communication between nerve cells so that the brain cannot function properly. The condition develops insidiously and the first problems noticed are usually related to memory loss. The old person may, for example, lose his way when he goes to the shops, or may mislay some of his belongings. If this is combined with a rather suspicious personality, accusations that someone has stolen these belongings may result. The old person may not remember what year and month it is, and eventually may even forget his own address. In the advanced stage of the disease, even familiar friends and relatives may not be identified and the person may try to leave his own house, not realising that he is at home. This often represents a regression to childhood and, when questioned, the old person will sometimes admit that he is trying to go back to his parents' address. As the condition progresses, relatives and friends can become frustrated because they seem to be unable to communicate with the old person who will either not listen to them or, if he does listen, will quickly forget what has been said.

If the old person with brain damage sees a situation differently from others in the same environment, he may become very unco-operative. He may argue with those who try to persuade him to look after his personal cleanliness because he wrongly believes that he has just had a bath. An elderly female with memory loss may fight with nurses who try to prevent her from leaving the ward, because she believes she has got to get home to feed the baby. Some demented people become particularly restless and seem to have a compulsion to wander off. This is particularly difficult when it occurs at night. Constantly disturbed sleep is one of the problems which relatives find most difficult to cope with. As the disease progresses, the sufferer may become unable to dress himself or perform other simple tasks of self-care and, ultimately, may lose the ability to control bowel and bladder, and may need to be fed.

Three remarks are necessary to qualify this rather gloomy picture. Firstly, many old people suffer a degree of benign memory loss which is not followed by the deterioration detailed here. Secondly, dementia is a disorder which progresses at quite different rates in different people and, although some may deteriorate rapidly, others may only deteriorate very gradually. Thirdly, all the problems of behaviour mentioned may be exacerbated by other factors, so that, while the underlying disease is irreversible, the associated behavioural disorders are sometimes amenable to psychiatric and psychological treatment.

Senile dementia may be mimicked by other conditions, including Vitamin B12 and thyroid deficiencies. For this reason, a careful medical assessment, early in the course of the disease, is essential. It is important that the doctor should know the history of the condition, in order to arrive at the correct diagnosis, and he or she usually questions relatives or close friends about the time course of the development of the illness. The patient's mental state needs to be assessed, too, in order that any necessary physical examinations and laboratory investigations can be carried out. In addition, the doctor will be interested in the amount of social support the old person is receiving, and whether any modifications can be made to this, in order to minimise disability and reduce the pressure on relatives and other helpers.

When a person is physically handicapped, many technological aids can be used to help them to cope. For example, a person who is almost paralysed can still operate a call system for nursing care, and may even be able to read books and do a constructive job with suitable technical help. However, a person who is demented gradually loses the ability to regulate his or her own environment. In the early stages of dementia, intermittent support may be sufficient to keep a person alive and well. However, as the disease progresses, the sufferer becomes less and less able to look after himself, and intermittent care becomes inappropriate. At the point where a 24-hour surveillance is required, full-time care in the home of the family, or in an old people's home, becomes essential. Some relatives are unaware of social services, such as meals on wheels, home helps, day centres and 'granny-sitting' services, or of how to obtain them. Putting caring relatives in contact with such services, and planning the care network so that the burden is shared between relatives, friends and social services, can improve the quality of life for both relatives and patient, and avoid unnecessary admission to hospital.

Another fairly common form of dementia in old age is due to the blood supply to small areas of the brain being cut off. This results in the death (infarction) of these areas of the brain, and when sufficient of these lesions accumulate, the behavioural changes of dementia emerge. Because of the way this form of dementia is caused, it is often called multi-infarct dementia (MID), or sometimes vascular or arteriosclerotic dementia. Untreated high blood pressure can contribute to this disorder, and it is to be hoped that, with improved medical control of blood pressure, the number of people suffering from multi-infarct dementia will decline.

Although the overall picture is much the same as in senile dementia, there are certain differences. The onset can be quite sudden, probably corresponding to the death of a small area of brain. The course of the condition, rather than being a gradual decline, tends to consist of a series of steps, when the patient is stable for a period of time, and then suddenly deteriorates, often with a partial recovery. Figure 3 gives a schematic outline of the different time courses of senile dementia of the Alzheimer type (SDAT), and of multi-infarct dementia (MID). As brain damage is rather patchy, the patient's mental state may be patchy, too, and he may be more aware of memory problems and more frustrated than when damage is more global. He may be unable to control his emotions and switch rapidly from being happy to being very sad, although the predominant mood is depression. Occasionally, explosive outbursts of anger may occur. Sometimes, there can be physical signs of stroke illness. Unlike SDAT, MID is more common in men and in the relatively young elderly. Although

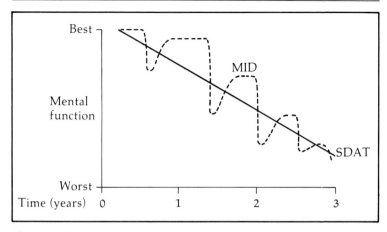

Fig. 3 A schematic presentation of the different time courses of senile dementia of the Alzheimer type (SDAT), and of multi-infarct dementia (MID).

the differentiation between senile dementia of the Alzheimer type and multi-infarct dementia is largely academic at present, as medical research progresses one or other of these conditions may become treatable.

Standardised scales are available for assessing memory and behaviour. Two of these are produced in Fig. 4. They form a useful basis for assessing change, and, in the case of the behavioural scale for identifying problem areas, it is useful for nurses and others looking after demented people to use these scales habitually, as they form a relatively objective measure of change.

Functional disorders

These fall into two main groups, the 'affective' illnesses, characterised by a predominant disturbance of mood, and the 'schizophrenic' illnesses, characterised by disturbances of thinking, hallucinations and delusions, often of a persecutory nature. Affective disorders commonly take the form of recurrent episodes of severe depression. Sometimes an elevated mood and overactivity are seen in the same person, often alternating with

Fig. 4 Two standardised scales for assessing (*a*) memory and (*b*) behaviour.

Hodkinson memory information scale

1. Age ......
2. Time (to nearest hour) ......
3. Address for recall at end of test ......
4. Year ......
5. Name of hospital

6. Recognition of two people ......
7. Date of birth ......
8. Years of First World War ......
9. Name of present monarch ......
10. Count backwards (20-1) ......

Modified Crichton Royal behavioural rating scale

Mobility:
0. Fully ambulant including stairs.
1. Usually independent.
2. Walks with minimum supervision.
3. Walks with aids or under close supervision.
4. Bedfast or chairfast.

☐

Orientation:
0. Complete.
1. Orientated in ward, identifies persons correctly.
2. Misidentifies persons but can find way about.
3. Cannot find way to bed or toilet without assistance.
4. Completely lost.

☐

Communication:
0. Always clear, retains information.
1. Can indicate needs, understands verbal directions and can deal with simple information.
2. Understands simple information, but cannot indicate needs.
3. Cannot understand information, but retains expressive ability.
4. No effective contact.

☐

Co-operation:
0. Actively co-operative.
1. Passively co-operative.
2. Requires frequent encouragement or persuasion.
3. Rejects assistance and shows independent ill-directed activity.
4. Completely resistive or withdrawn.

☐

Restlessness:
0. None.
1. Intermittent.
2. Persistent by day or night.
3. Persistent by day and night.
4. Constant.

☐

Dressing:
0. Correct.
1. Imperfect but adequate.
2. Adequate with minimum supervision.
3. Inadequate unless continually supervised.
4. Unable to dress or to retain clothing.

☐

Feeding:
0. Correct unaided at appropriate times.
1. Adequate with minimum of supervision.
2. Inadequate unless continually supervised.
3. Requires feeding.

☐

Continence:
0. Full control.
1. Occasional accidents.
2. Continent by day only if regularly toiletted.
3. Urinary incontinence in spite of regular toiletting.
4. Regular or frequent double incontinence.

☐

episodes of depression. These elevated episodes are referred to as 'hypomania'. Old people who have been subject to attacks of recurrent depression in earlier life often have further attacks in old age. Sometimes they develop hypomania for the first time, thus breaking a lifetime pattern of recurrent depressive illness. Severe depressive illness may arise for the first time in old age, although careful enquiry can reveal a previous history of untreated depressive episodes, or that someone else in the family has suffered from depressive illness.

Like many words in psychiatry, 'depression' has different shades of meaning. It is used to describe the feeling some people have on a Monday morning. It is used descriptively within psychiatry to refer to a disturbance of mood which may be present in many different psychiatric conditions. The use we are considering here is in the term 'depressive illness' or 'depressive psychosis' where it is attached to a definite pattern of experience and behaviour which is medically recognized and usually amenable to treatment. Depressive illness develops usually over a period of weeks or months, and commonly starts with a loss of interest and withdrawal from the outside world. The sufferer may begin to neglect his appearance and personal hygiene and may find that tasks which were previously easy become burdensome. The patient usually describes his feelings as unhappy or miserable, although severely depressed patients may complain of feeling 'nothing' at all. Thoughts and speech tend to become morbidly preoccupied with concern about bodily health, or imaginary or overstated guilt, or poverty. Sometimes, thought processes and behaviour slow down markedly, and the sufferer becomes unable to reach decisions, even about quite simple matters. In other cases he will become agitated and may make frequent importunate requests for reassurance from helpers. Sleep is disturbed and appetite often reduced.

If a patient is very depressed, he may develop firm convictions that he has committed some unforgivable sin, or that he is suffering from an untreatable illness. These are called depressive delusions. Hallucinatory voices, accusing the patient of wrong doing or making derogatory remarks, may be heard and usually are felt by the patient to be justified. The patient often underestimates his own capabilities and may complain of failing memory. Indeed, on formal memory-testing, some depressed patients do very poorly, but this is usually a result, rather than a cause, of the depression, and, when the depressive illness is treated, the memory tends to improve. The patient may reach the point where he feels that life is no longer worth living, and may wish to commit suicide. Elderly depressed men living alone are particularly at risk of suicide, especially if they have been bereaved recently. The risk of suicide should be borne in mind, therefore, when dealing with elderly depressed people.

Severe depression needs treatment with medication or with electroconvulsive therapy. Sometimes the patient can be treated as an outpatient, but admission to hospital, either as an inpatient or day patient, can be necessary. Although electroconvulsive therapy (ECT) has received a rather 'bad press', there is no doubt that, in properly selected patients, it is very effective in alleviating severe depression. In many old people the main problem is not treating the acute episode of depression, but preventing recurrence. Medication can be helpful but measures to increase social support and widen the range of social contact are also important. In addition, some patients respond to psychological treatments, either in individual, or group, psychotherapy, which is designed to help them cope with the problems of old age and to develop a more positive attitude towards themselves and the difficulties of ageing. When a person is severely depressed, it is no use telling him to 'snap out of it' as he will not be able to, and his very inability may cause him to become even more depressed. As the patient begins to recover from his depression, he can be encouraged gradually to take more responsibility for himself and helped to form a more positive image of himself.

Hypomanic states are rare in old age. In these, the patient becomes over-active, excitable and may spend money recklessly. In old people, the mood is often a mixture of elation with some depressed feelings. Like severely depressed patients, patients with hypomania often have little insight into their illness, and compulsory treatment in hospital can be necessary, and is usually successful.

The main form of schizophrenic illness in old age is called 'late paraphrenia'. This can develop in a predisposed personality. The characteristic sufferer is an unmarried elderly lady who has been socially isolated and who develops the conviction that she is being persecuted, or attacked sexually, in the absence of any external cause. This kind of false, unshakeable belief is called a delusion. In addition, there may be false perceptions (hallucinations) in which the person hears voices talking about her or in which she feels she is being touched or otherwise molested, again in the absence of any external stimulus. In their more florid form, these conditions demand treatment with drugs from the group known as 'major tranquillisers', and hospital admission is often necessary. Usually treatment is remarkably successful and the person can return to his own home. Sometimes, fortnightly, or even monthly, injections of long-acting drugs are all that is needed to maintain health. There are other conditions in which persecutory delusions are experienced, perhaps the commonest being dementia complicated by persecutory delusions. When a patient is deluded, it is no use arguing with him; however, if the helper does not agree with the patient's delusions, it will be helpful if he or she appreciates that they are 'real' to the patient.

Neurotic disorders and personality

Neurotic disorders occur when a person has developed ways of dealing with stress that are 'maladaptive' in the sense that they cause more problems than they solve. Excessive anxiety, either 'free-floating' (anxiety state) or attached to particular objects (phobias), obsessions, and some mild forms of depression, are examples of neurotic disorders. These may have been a life-long pattern or may emerge for the first time in old age in response to the special stresses of ageing in our society. Generally speaking, they are best not treated with drugs and, if they are causing problems, can often best be dealt with by counselling or psychotherapeutic means, including behaviour therapy. Negative personality traits can be exacerbated in depressive illness, but become less prominent when the illness is treated effectively.

Alcohol and drug abuse is not as rare in old age as is commonly assumed. Some life-long alcoholics survive into old age, and others start to abuse alcohol for the first time in response to the stresses of ageing. Excessive alcohol or drug consumption in old people should not be regarded as a harmless foible but as a potentially damaging disorder requiring appropriate medical and social help. Some elderly heavy drinkers depend on others to provide their alcohol and sometimes have several suppliers who are unknown to each other.

In some families, unhelpful interactions between members can produce severe problems. These include physical attacks by one member of the family on another. Sometimes the old person is the aggressor; sometimes the victim. On other occasions, the problem may be that an elderly ailing mother complains of her problems to her child, who spends more and more time with the old lady, which produces marital or other problems within the family. Often these problems have simple roots in the way the people in the family habitually respond to one another.

A woman who had been in a mental hospital with chronic depression was discharged after treatment. She lived alone, but was always asking her son to come round, constantly asking for his help when it was not really necessary, and saying: 'What do I do?' She was also shouting a great deal, which was disturbing the neighbours, and was doing very little for herself in the house. She complained of loneliness and it was noteworthy that her ability to look after herself was much better when she attended the day hospital. After careful assessment of the situation, the son agreed to participate in a programme of psychological management. He agreed not to do things for her which she could do for herself, and to tell her that he thought she could manage to do these things. He also agreed to reduce the time he spent with her if she started to shout and, with the help of the psychologist, set gradually increasing goals for self-care. When she achieved these goals, he rewarded her by spending more time with her.

Her capabilities in the day hospital were demonstrated to the son who was told not to criticise her for not doing so well at home, but to concentrate on praising her when she achieved something. Her functioning steadily improved, and her shouting became much less troublesome. The son spends less time with her and she receives less criticism from the neighbours, now that they are relieved of her shouting. The situation, which could have resulted in great distress for both son and mother, and in her being unnecessarily removed to a long-stay hospital, was thus coped with by careful application of basic psychological principles.

PHYSICAL HEALTH AND NUTRITION

Prolonged physical ill health can produce a depressive reaction. Sometimes this can be dealt with best by discussing the illness frankly with the patient and encouraging him to find ways to compensate for his disabilities. In other cases, physical illness may precipitate a depressive illness which should be treated in its own right. When depression and physical illness co-exist, special care must be taken in the choice of medication, but it is important to ensure that the depression is treated adequately as this may produce more disability than the underlying physical illness.

Physical illness can precipitate an acute confusional state (delirium). The patient may be well preserved mentally or may be suffering from a degree of dementia. A physical illness, such as heart failure, a chest infection or a urinary infection, causes the sudden onset of severe confusion. In addition to the features found in dementia, the patient may have vivid auditory and visual hallucinations and is often extremely frightened by his experiences. This fear may give rise to violent behaviour if the patient is not handled correctly. Acute confusional states tend to be worse in the evening. Whilst the underlying condition is being treated, the patient should be sedated, if necessary. He should be nursed in a well-lit room, preferably by people who are familiar to him. Great care should be taken to reassure him, and remind him where he is and who the people are who are trying to help him. Such reassurance will help the patient to retain contact with reality and prevent disturbed behaviour. A well known form of acute confusional state is delirium tremens (DTs) which occurs when alcohol is withdrawn from someone who has become dependent on it. It is not unknown in old people and should be suspected when an unexplained acute confusional state develops a few days after admission to hospital or a residential home. If a history of excessive alcohol intake is proved, delirium tremens can be prevented during alcohol withdrawal by the use of appropriate medication.

The elderly alcoholic is often poorly nourished and may be deficient in thiamine. Deficiency of this vitamin can cause an acute confusional state with double vision and unsteadiness on the feet called 'Wernicke's encephalopathy', which may, in turn, lead to the permanent memory loss or 'Korsakoff's psychosis'. Although this condition is relatively rare, it is very important because it can be prevented by the intravenous administration of a thiamine-containing preparation. Elderly patients who do not abuse alcohol may also be relatively low in thiamine, and the use of vitamin supplements during acute illness, or following an accident, may well be important in reducing the risks of confusion. Poor nutrition may be secondary to mental illness and self-neglect. Folic acid deficiency commonly accompanies dementia when the patient lives alone and does not take adequate meals. The depressed patient may fail to eat and drink to the point where this becomes life-threatening. This can be regarded as a form of 'slow suicide' and demands urgent action.

DRUGS

Modern medications are extremely powerful and have brought great benefit to many old people. Nevertheless, they are probably over-prescribed for old people and, because of their potency, can cause considerable problems. Because of the risk of side-effects and because of the danger of interaction between different drugs, certain principles are important in prescribing and giving medication to elderly people. Firstly, a distinction must be made between the use of drugs to cure or alleviate specific illnesses, (such as the use of antidepressants for depressive illness), and the use of drugs simply to control symptoms (such as the use of powerful tranquillisers for the behaviourally disturbed demented patient or the use of sleeping tablets for someone who is not mentally ill, but complains of insomnia).

Secondly, alternatives to medication should be considered. For example, if an old person complains of lack of sleep, further enquiry should be made to determine the exact pattern of sleep disturbance. It may be a symptom of depressive illness, in which case the proper treatment is that of the underlying illness. On the other hand, the old person may be sleeping quite adequately but may have unrealistic expectations of how long he or she should sleep. Increased physical exercise during the day can improve night-time sleep, and 'cat-napping' during the day should be avoided if a good night's rest is wanted. When medication is needed, it should be prescribed in the smallest effective dose and treatment should not be continued beyond the time that is medically necessary. Care should be taken when more than one drug is prescribed as the possibility of interaction increases rapidly as more drugs are taken.

> A 70-year-old man, living with his wife, had had several episodes of heart trouble and had been put on to two drugs to control his heart rhythm. Perhaps partly as a consequence of this, he had become rather depressed and an antidepressant had been prescribed. This antidepressant interacted with the other drugs to cause a severe drop in blood pressure whenever the old man stood up. As a consequence, he became even more depressed and practically chair-bound. After being seen at home by the psychiatrist, he was taken into hospital by a geriatrician where all of his drugs were withdrawn and he gradually returned to good mental, and reasonable physical, health.

When old people are given drugs to take, it is important to make sure that they are in containers which the old person can open, with large-print labels, and that the purpose of the drug and the dosage regime is carefully explained. Fifteen minutes spent by doctor, nurse or pharmacist in explaining the patient's tablets is probably the best way of ensuring that the tablets are taken properly.

ETHICAL ISSUES

Mental illness in old age raises particular ethical problems because the patient's judgement can be impaired and others, therefore, have to take responsibility for him. In depressive illness, it may, for example, be necessary to admit someone to hospital on a compulsory order because of the risk of suicide. The demented patient may not be able to understand the implications of coming into hospital or moving into an old people's home, and decisions may have to be taken on his behalf. If necessary, the management of the patient's financial affairs can be taken over by a receiver under the Court of Protection, but the procedure for this is rather cumbersome and many demented old people's financial affairs are looked after by their relatives on an informal basis. Application to the Court of Protection is necessary if there is fear of exploitation, or if large sums of money are involved.

A practical issue often raised is whether or not to go along with the demented patient's perception of the world. If the demented patient insists on leaving the ward, is this best handled by confrontation, simply telling him that he cannot go, or by deceit – for example, telling him that the bus he needs to catch to go home can only be caught in the ward day room? In most cases, a third alternative – diversion – is the best policy. The situation just discussed might, for example, be dealt with by reminding the person that he is in hospital and that the nurses are nurses who want to help him, and by offering to have a cup of tea with him. This kind of diversion avoids both outright deceit and a potential confrontation.

A particular issue is how far severely demented patients should be treated if they develop a terminal illness. The medical decision here depends on individual circumstances, including the views of relatives and nurses and the certainty of the diagnosis. Measures of doubtful benefit which would cause pain or discomfort to the patient, or which merely prolong suffering, should be avoided. Ill-considered efforts to save life at any cost benefit nobody.

SERVICES

Specialist psychiatric services for the elderly are developing at an increasing rate. There are now over 120 consultant psychiatrists in the United Kingdom working specially with the elderly and, at the time of writing, more than half of them have come into this work within the past five years. However, many of the developing psychiatric services for old people are seriously under-resourced and cannot provide the full range of community, acute inpatient, day hospital and long-stay hospital places that should be available. Nevertheless, the development of the services, and their close collaboration with geriatric medical services and social services, is the key to adequate psychiatric care for old people. A full psychiatric assessment of the mentally ill elderly person, taking into account environmental factors, sensory problems, physical health and medication, as well as psychiatric illness, is essential. Continuing involvement by professions from different disciplines within the psychiatric team for the elderly can help maintain old people within the community, whether they are suffering from an irreversible mental illness, or have been treated for a reversible condition such as depression. An optimistic approach, which systematically reviews the various factors considered in Fig. 1, will result in the best possible quality of life for the mentally ill old person and will avoid the defeatist attitude that 'nothing can be done'.

Further reading

Those requiring further information on clinical aspects of the psychiatry of old age are referred to:

Pitt, Brice, *Psychogeriatrics* (Churchill Livingstone, 2nd edition, 1982).

A practical book for helpers is:

Keddie, *Action with the Elderly* (Pergamon, 1978).

4

DRUG THERAPY AND THE ELDERLY

DR CYRIL JOSEPHS

Senior Medical Officer,
Nightingale House, Home for Aged Jews,
Clapham, London

Approximately one person in eight of the population is over 65, yet this group accounts for one-third of the drug bill incurred by the National Health Service. The use of medicines of all kinds has become extremely prevalent in the community and people have come to expect tablets or medicine for almost any condition. The enormous number of drug preparations that is now available, and the expectancy of the patient or his relatives for tangible treatment from the doctor, has led to far more prescribing of potent drugs than hitherto. Twenty years ago the choice of drugs was more limited; patients were less well-informed and not subject to the wide publicity given to many medical matters by the newspapers, radio and television. There is no doubt that there have been great advances in the pharmaceutical field and these will continue.

However, with these advances and the emergence of ever-more potent drugs comes an increase in hazards: hazards due to undesirable side-effects of drugs and many due to undesirable interaction of different drugs. New preparations appear on the market with great frequency and, although these have been carefully tested before becoming available to the practising doctor, such tests have rarely been carried out on old people specifically. It is of great importance to realise that treatment of old people with drugs presents problems that are encountered less often in younger patients because the old frequently react differently. There are several reasons why such problems arise.

THE DISTRIBUTION OF DRUGS IN THE BODY

The composition of the body changes with age. There is often a reduction in lean tissue and an increase in body fat. This relative change can affect the fate of a fat-soluble drug, such as diazepam, which will tend therefore to accumulate in an old person, so producing a prolonged action. Put another way, it means that an old person will need less diazepam than his younger counterpart to produce a similar effect. Some drugs such as warfarin and phenylbutazone become bound to protein and are inactive when so bound. Since sick old people have less protein in the blood (serum albumin) the amount of unbound (active) drug may increase. Again this means that a lower dose of the drug is needed.

METABOLISM

Most drugs are metabolised in the liver, after which they become inactive and are excreted in the bile or in the urine. The rate at which the metabolism breakdown occurs determines the amount of active drug present in the body, and consequently its duration of action. Liver function diminishes in old age and consequently increases the time a drug remains active.

RENAL EXCRETION

Effective renal function decreases with age. It has been estimated that, when people reach the age of 40 and over, the function declines by approximately 1 per cent per year. Thus the glomerular filtration rate in a man of 75 will be approximately 65 per cent of that of a young adult. This is readily seen by the raised urea and creatinine so often found in the serum of old people.

This decreased renal function will prolong the active life of a drug. This is usually disadvantageous, as in the case of digoxin, which easily causes toxicity. Sometimes there will be an advantage, for example with some antibiotics, but even then the liability to unpleasant reactions is increased. Some antibiotics have profound toxic effects above a fairly critical level. Examples of these are streptomycin and gentamicin, which have a narrow margin of safety that makes them more dangerous for old people.

INCREASED TISSUE SENSITIVITY

In the elderly, increased sensitivity of the target organs occurs frequently and this is a potent cause of side-effects, since the drug effectiveness is frequently enhanced. Untoward symptoms include not only those which are relatively common in young adults, but also some which are less well-known. Most problems occur with diuretics, digoxin, antidepressants, tranquillisers, hypnotics, rigidity controllers, steroids and hypotensives. It must be remembered that all of these drugs are important, useful, and sometimes life-saving. It must also be remembered that any drug will have potential side-effects unless it is quite inert and that old people are particularly sensitive. There are many unwanted effects of drugs: the symptoms most commonly encountered are shown in Table 5.

Table 5 The unwanted side-effects of some drugs

Symptom	Drugs frequently implicated
Anorexia	Digoxin, levodopa.
Cardiac arrhythmia	Digoxin, tricyclic antidepressants.
Confusion	Digoxin, anti-Parkinsonian drugs, tricyclic antidepressants, phenothiazines, betablockers, sedatives, cortico-steroids.
Constipation	Morphine, diamorphine, codeine.
Depression	Levodopa, methyldopa, reserpine, barbiturates, indomethacin.
Diabetes mellitus	Thiazide diuretics, cortico-steroids.
Diarrhoea	Broad spectrum antibiotics, magnesium trisilicate.
Gastrointestinal bleeding	Aspirin, phenylbutazone, indomethacin, cortico-steroids.
Gout	Thiazide diuretics.
Hypokalaemia (low potassium)	Diuretics.
Hyponatraemia (low sodium)	Diuretics, chlorpropamide.
Hypotension (low blood pressure), a frequent cause of falls	Phenothiazines, tricyclic antidepressants, anti-hypertensive drugs.
Hypothermia (low body heat)	Phenothiazines, barbiturates.
Involuntary movements (dyskinesia)	Phenothiazines, levodopa.
Jaundice	Anabolic-steroids, phenothiazines.
Parkinsonism	Phenothiazines.
Skin rashes	Many drugs – especially broad spectrum antibiotics.
Urinary incontinence	Diuretics, hypnotics.

While it is important not to withhold treatment because a patient is old, one has to be constantly on the alert for possible side-effects, which are so much more common than in young people. Doses given usually will be smaller than those advised normally. When a fresh symptom develops soon after starting a new medication, it is as well to suspect the new treatment: the diagnosis will often be correct. This is particularly true of confusion and depression, the symptoms of which are not infrequently directly due to drugs. It is easy and all too common for further drugs to be added to alleviate the new symptoms, thus compounding the problem. Often one sees an elderly patient with multiple symptoms in whom the original complaint is overshadowed, or completely hidden, by the overlay of iatrogenic symptoms. Only by stopping most or all of the drugs can the physician reveal the real organic symptoms, if any exist.

THE PROBLEM OF COMPLIANCE

All too often elderly patients have considerable difficulty understanding what seem to be quite straightforward drug regimes. The habit of treating each fresh symptom with an additional drug frequently results in a total daily dose which is quite ludicrous. It is by no means uncommon for the total number of tablets taken daily to exceed a dozen; even a young person would be daunted by the treatment advised. Repeat prescriptions are often given without the doctor seeing the patient, and without his appraising the situation properly to check which drugs should, or should not, be continued.

While it is generally undesirable to give compound tablets, that is tablets which contain two or more active ingredients which prevent the dose of individual components being altered separately, a good case can be made for giving such compound tablets to old people whenever possible. This policy will lessen the number of tablets needed daily and make compliance more likely. Some preparations are available in slow release form and can thus be given once daily.

The elderly often have difficulty in getting their tablets out of the containers. Many of the child-proof containers (which have certainly lessened the number of cases of accidental poisoning in children) are adult-proof, too, particularly when the adult has poor eyesight or arthritic fingers. Of those with adequate eyesight and no finger deformities, one recent survey showed that almost a third were quite unable to get at their drugs. However, many elderly patients do require a number of different medicines and the efficacy of their self-medication will depend largely on the manner of their presentation.

Instruction labels printed in large type are a great help to the poorlysighted. Various dispensing aids have been developed. The 'Dosett' box (Penmill Limited) contains 28 compartments and can hold up to one week's supply of drugs taken four times daily. If the patient goes out for the day he must take the whole week's supply with him. The 'Medidos' system consists of seven separate rectangular compartments, one for each day of the week, each of which is divided by three movable dividers separating the daily dose into four, i.e. breakfast, lunch, tea and supper. Each rectangular compartment contains one day's supply of tablets and can be taken separately by the patient if on a day's outing. With either the 'Dosett' or the 'Medidos' box, the week's supply has to be inserted by the nurse, doctor or those in attendance. Errors are reduced when using these boxes, but care is needed in order to avoid spillage between the compartments. Drugs missed on previous days must *not* be taken all at once. No ploy is completely successful and the patient who has constant help at hand is the most fortunate. The doctor can help considerably by anticipating these problems and by keeping the number of tablets prescribed as low as possible, taking into account the amount of assistance available.

SOME DRUGS THAT ARE COMMONLY PRESCRIBED

Diuretics

The introduction of oral diuretics revolutionised the treatment of oedema, whether from cardiac, renal, or liver disease. The commonest of these is cardiac oedema and the coupling of digoxin therapy with adequate diuresis allows the distressing symptoms of cardiac failure to be controlled more readily. When the failure affects mainly the left side of the heart (left ventricular failure), pulmonary oedema with severe breathlessness (cardiac asthma) occurs, often in the early hours of the morning. Diuretics can bring profound relief of symptoms and are a real boon to the sufferer. They should not be given at night, except in an emergency. This commonly prescribed group of drugs can cause numerous problems and side-effects. The more important of these are electrolyte disturbances, urinary incontinence, falls due to hypotension, gout and hyperglycaemia. The drugs should be given for clear-cut reasons, and discontinued as soon as possible. The serum electrolytes should be monitored and potassium supplements are frequently needed. Occasionally, sodium supplements are required.

Hypnotics

Hypnotics are undoubtedly prescribed too often and for too long. Sleeplessness needs confirming since many old people complain that they are awake all night when this is often not corroborated by those in attendance. Some sleep periodically during the day and can hardly be expected to sleep all night too. Insomnia, due to pain, a troubled mind, a stuffy room, or a full bladder, needs attention to the cause, and not the prescription of a hypnotic. Insomnia may be a manifestation of depression which requires antidepressants. When a sedative is prescribed (and it is sometimes justified) it should be a relatively short-acting drug and one with a wide margin of safety. Chloral is useful and can be given in tablet form which lessens the incidence of gastric irritation. Chlormethiazole and shorter-acting benzodiazepines – lormetazepam or temazepam – have relatively less hangover effect, and are relatively safe.

Patients tend to develop tolerance to hypnotics after two or three weeks and to develop dependence after a longer period, making withdrawal more difficult. Barbiturates should not be used in the elderly because of the frequent undesirable side-effects, not the least of which are hypotension, confusion and dependence.

Tranquillisers

These present similar problems to the hypnotics and many belong to the same group of drugs. If a benzodiazepine is needed, a short-acting one, such as lorazepam, is preferable to the longer-acting diazepam, though undue sensitivity is not infrequent.

The major tranquillisers can be useful when agitation is prominent but all have unpleasant side-effects and are particularly likely to cause Parkinsonism, which can develop after only a few tablets have been taken, and persist long after they have been stopped. Thioridazine is popular for treating the elderly, as there is less likelihood of side-effects. Hypnotics and tranquillisers potentiate the effect of alcohol, and patients or relatives should be made aware of this.

Laxatives

There is no justification nowadays for the use of strong laxatives and purgatives in the elderly. A faecal softener, such as lactulose, should be effective in preventing hard stools, but a loaded colon may have to be cleared first by a series of enemas given daily for three to seven days. (An oral preparation of standardised senna is useful.) Sometimes bisacodyl suppositories will obviate the need for an enema.

There is no justification for taking a laxative daily for several years, but this is not uncommon in the elderly. It is surprising how the need for the daily dose can vanish without mishap soon after admission to hospital. It is also surprising how often the patient reverts to his habit soon after returning home.

Antidepressants

These are very useful drugs and are commonly prescribed. Tricyclics (e.g. amitriptyline and imipramine) and the newer tetracyclics (e.g. mianserin) are relatively safe, but should be started in small doses. They can cause annoying constipation, dryness of the mouth, and cardiac arrhythmia.

Hypotensives

Drugs used to lower blood pressure are prescribed frequently, but at present hypertension is generally treated less energetically in the elderly. This is probably a wise policy, since the treatment is frequently more unpleasant than the disease. However, there is some evidence that keeping blood pressure at 160/100 mmHg or below, lessens the chances of long-term sequelae. Diuretics are probably the best first-line treatment, after which a cardio-selective beta blocker, such as atenolol, can be added, if needed. Small doses should be used at first as postural hypotension is a definite risk, with the consequent hazard of a fall on rising from bed. It is not acceptable to exchange a symptomless hypertension for a fractured femur.

Drugs for Parkinson's disease

There is no doubt that the discovery of levodopa has helped many old people with this very distressing and disabling condition, even though the benefit seems to diminish after about two years. The drug frequently causes nausea and loss of appetite but combining levodopa with carbidopa causes far fewer problems and can improve rigidity and slowness quite remarkably. Anticholinergic drugs used for Parkinsonism reduce tremor and rigidity, and are a useful adjunct to dopamine. Unfortunately they can cause confusion and can precipitate glaucoma and urinary retention.

Digoxin

This drug is very beneficial when rapid atrial fibrillation exists, particularly if heart failure with oedema coexists. It is less effective when cardiac rhythm is regular. It should be given in small doses; rarely is more than 0.25 mg required daily. Many patients can be stabilised on 0.0625 mg daily, a dose which was formulated with old people in mind. Digoxin has a narrow therapeutic range and toxicity is common. It slows the heart very effectively, but has the unfortunate habit of increasing the rate when at a high toxic level in the blood. This tachycardia may mislead the physician, who increases the dose, so compounding the problem. It is now common and good practice to estimate the content of digoxin in the blood, which should be kept below 2 ng/ml. Apart from its effect on the heart, digoxin frequently causes confusion, nausea, vomiting, diarrhoea or a cardiac arrhythmia. Toxicity is more common nowadays since diuretics are so often prescribed. These may lower the tissue potassium, which in turn renders the myocardium more sensitive to digoxin.

It is not sufficiently appreciated that elderly people taking digoxin need not always continue the drug for life, and it is important to review the situation at regular intervals. The correct dose is that which is needed to keep the heart rate normal; often the digoxin can be discontinued after several weeks. It can always be reintroduced if the indications for it recur.

Analgesics

The underlying cause of pain should be treated, where possible, rather than the pain itself. Despite this bland statement, analgesics are required, either while the cause of the pain is being treated, or because no effective treatment is available for the primary condition. When pain disturbs sleep, its relief by adequate analgesia will be more effective than heavy sedation.

Musculoskeletal pain is common in the elderly and can be distressing and disabling. Mild analgesics, with or without anti-inflammatory properties, are the drugs of first choice. Paracetamol is of low toxicity in ordinary doses, but it is of low potency. Giving two tablets three times daily may be effective. Aspirin remains a most useful analgesic and is best given in soluble form. A compound of paracetamol and dextropropoxyphene (e.g. distalgesic) is popular and often more effective than aspirin or paracetamol, but one wonders how much of the benefit accrues from its distinctive and attractive shape and marking. Newer analgesics are appearing on the market constantly, but the manufacturers' claims are by no means always borne out in practice.

Some common side-effects of the milder analgesics

Aspirin

Aspirin often causes occult gastrointestinal bleeding, with resultant anaemia. It is best taken after meals. It may potentiate oral hypoglycaemic drugs (of the sulphonylurea group) and anti-coagulants such as warfarin. It has to be discontinued occasionally because of sensitivity reactions (skin rashes, facial oedema, tinnitus and wheezing).

Paracetamol and dextropropoxyphene compound

This seems to cause confusion in some, and dizziness, nausea and constipation are not uncommon.

Pentazocine

This is more potent than aspirin or paracetamol, but can cause clouding of consciousness, and even hallucinations.

The fenamates

The fenamates (such as ibuprofen and ketoprofen) are used in rheumatic disorders, but the effectiveness is uncertain and side-effects are constantly being reported. It is likely that in time their usefulness will be assessed more accurately.

Indomethacin and phenylbutazone

These are best reserved for those with severe painful arthritis, since they can cause nausea, vomiting, confusion, fluid retention and, occasionally, dangerous bone-marrow suppression. Indomethacin occasionally causes hypersensitivity reactions, such as skin rashes, angioneurotic oedema (swelling of the face), or troublesome bronchospasm.

RELIEF OF PAIN IN THE DYING

It is imperative to relieve pain in the dying patient, and the fear of side-effects and dependency should be of no import. It is vital to give adequate doses of the more powerful analgesics. An adequate dose is the smallest which relieves the pain completely. The dose should be repeated at frequent enough intervals to anticipate pain recurring.

Morphine is still the most useful of the strong analgesics. It is well absorbed by mouth and reaches its peak blood level in between one-and-a-half to two hours. It is conveniently given in a mixture with chloroform water, or can be added to pro-chlorperazine syrup if nausea is troublesome. Nausea is not uncommon at the start of morphine treatment; it usually wears off after a few days. If and when pain is escaping control by the milder analgesics, oral morphine (5 to 10 mg) should be given every four hours. The dose can be increased after one or two days, if necessary. It should be given more frequently if pain is severe. By increasing the frequency or the strength of the dose, or both, complete freedom from pain, without undue sedation, is possible.

Analgesic injections are rarely needed simply to control pain, but will be essential if the patient cannot swallow, is vomiting persistently, or is semicomatose. Morphine is about twice as potent by injection as by mouth so half the effective oral dose should be sufficient. Diamorphine is similar to morphine by mouth, but, being more soluble, can be given by injection in a smaller volume. Alternative powerful analgesics include dex-tromoramide, dipipanone, methadone and phenazocine. Each has its advocates.

The patient dying in pain is anathema and it is inexcusable that someone in this predicament should be denied whatever dose at whatever frequency is required to bring relief. Contrary to popular belief (even today), the dosage required is often quite small, does not increase and does not necessarily shorten life. Efficient pain relief may prolong life; it certainly improves the quality of dying.

The invention of a battery-operated syringe which gives a measured subcutaneous dose at regular intervals is very useful in selected cases and allows a degree of mobility to such patients hitherto undreamed of.

POINTS TO REMEMBER

It is important that the following points are borne in mind when prescribing drugs for the elderly:

1. Too many old people take too many drugs for too long.
2. The indications for and the benefits of discontinuing drugs are at least as profound as for their initiation.
3. Most unsupervised elderly patients will make serious errors in their drug therapy if they are prescribed more than two drugs daily.
4. Accurate treatment depends on accurate diagnosis.
5. Try not to make the treatment worse than the disease.

6. Review a drug regime at frequent intervals.
7. Regularly ask the question: 'Does this patient still need this drug?'
8. Prescribe the smallest dose necessary. Half the recommended adult dose is a wise beginning.
9. If in doubt whether a drug is needed, it usually is not.
10. If an elderly patient becomes suddenly confused after starting a new drug, suspect the drug and stop it.

Postscript

An elderly housebound lady was visited routinely every month by her doctor who repeated her prescription for various drugs and checked how she was progressing and how she was coping with her various infirmities. This regular, conscientious visiting went on for several years until the old lady died peacefully. After her death, huge numbers of tablets of all shapes, sizes and colours were found in her flat. One is driven to the inescapable conclusion that the patient enjoyed the doctor's visits more than the tablets and felt that failure to accept the monthly prescription might curtail his visits. For his part, the doctor was convinced that his tablets were keeping his patient well, not realising what the really effective agent was. Both patient and doctor were happy.

5

NURSING CARE OF THE ELDERLY

SHEILA BAILEY

Clinical Tutor, Continuing and In-Service Education,
School of Nursing,
Addenbrooke's Hospital, Cambridge

In recent years a major change has taken place in the way nursing care is organised. Hitherto the reasons for the delivery of nursing care, which was provided in a very routine way, depended on the medical diagnosis; that is, all patients with the same disease, or undergoing similar operations, received virtually the same nursing care, irrespective of their individual differences. Now, increasingly, nursing care is planned to meet each patient's individual needs; what is considered is not the disease itself, but the effect the disease has on each person individually.

A system called the 'nursing process' has been introduced which puts nursing care on a more methodical basis. The process followed is in four stages as follows:
1. *Assessing* the patient's individual needs.
2. *Planning* the specific nursing care appropriate to his needs.
3. *Implementing* the plan by giving the nursing care.
4. *Evaluating* the effects of the care given, in order to see if it has achieved its objectives, and altering or adapting the plan of care as necessary.

The first stage of assessing the patient's needs is, of course, vitally important, and great emphasis has been laid in this section of the book on the need to observe and question the patient carefully, from the start, in order to identify all his problems accurately and comprehensively. If this stage is carried out thoroughly and objectively, an effective plan of care can be based on the findings.

A basic pattern or framework for assessment is needed, and a very practical framework has been laid down by a distinguished nurse tutor, Nancy Roper, in her book, *Elements of Nursing*. She sees the purpose of nursing as 'to preserve so far as possible the patient's usual habits and routines associated with each activity of living', and 'to help patients with particular problems related to activities of living'.

It is on Miss Roper's approach that this chapter on nursing care is based. She identified 12 activities of living, as follows:

1. Maintaining a safe environment.
2. Communicating.
3. Breathing.
4. Eating and drinking.
5. Eliminating waste products.
6. Personal cleansing and dressing.
7. Controlling body temperature.
8. Being mobile.
9. Working and playing.
10. Expressing sexuality.
11. Sleeping.
12. Dying.

Those activities appropriate to nursing care of the aged patient have been selected. Discussion of each activity will include an explanation of how it changes with advancing age, and how the deficiencies that commonly occur may be corrected or coped with.

BREATHING
The mechanism of breathing

The act of breathing brings oxygen in the air into close contact with the blood. This contact occurs in the lungs; from there the oxygen is carried, in the blood, to the heart and then pumped to all the cells of the body. Oxygen is essential to the life of all cells, especially the brain; without it a person would rapidly lose consciousness and die. Air is drawn in through the nose and mouth, through the larynx or voice box, into a network of branching tubes. These tubes get progressively smaller in diameter and end in minute balloon-like air sacs. It is through the thin walls of these air sacs that oxygen passes into the circulating blood. When we breathe in (inspiration) a large muscle, the diaphragm (which forms the floor of the chest), goes down, while muscles between the ribs pull the rib cage upwards and outwards, causing the elastic lungs to expand, drawing air into them. Breathing out (expiration) is the reverse of this process; the diaphragm moves up and the muscles between the ribs relax, pulling them down. The lungs are squeezed, forcing air out. The air passages produce a sticky substance which gathers up small particles that enter with the air. Small hair-like projections lining the air passages trap this debris. Their motion propels it out of the lungs and it is either swallowed or coughed out.

As a result of the ageing process, the lungs lose their elasticity and appear to be larger. The air sacs become fewer in number and larger in size. Consequently the amount of oxygen passing into the blood is reduced. The diaphragm and the muscles between the ribs become progressively weaker, so that the amount of air moved in and out of the lungs is reduced, and thus the amount of available oxygen is also reduced. Coughing also becomes more difficult; in addition, the action of the hair-like projections is decreased. This, and the interference with coughing, leads to an accumulation of the sticky secretions in the air passages. Thus the elderly are more prone to respiratory problems and infections.

The heart is a muscular organ and its function is to pump blood around the body, and to the lungs, through a system of arteries and veins. The main functions of the blood are to transport oxygen, nutrients and other important substances to the cells of the body, and to take waste products from the cells to various organs in the body to be eliminated. As one grows older the pumping efficiency of the heart is reduced. Blood vessels lose their elasticity and become thickened, and this results in a rise in blood pressure. The changes in the heart and blood vessels mean that the delivery of oxygen and nutrients to cells is less efficient and the functioning of all the organs of the body is reduced. The changes in blood vessels and the raised blood pressure make elderly people more prone to such diseases as strokes and heart failure. Some of the breathing problems that affect elderly people are caused by the degenerative changes in the heart and blood vessels.

Assessment of breathing
1. Cough

Coughing is an important, protective mechanism. A person with respiratory problems, such as an infection, may have a persistent cough. The first thing to notice about the cough is, when does it occur? It is not uncommon for elderly people to cough first thing in the morning when they get up. If the cough continues after this, and during sleep, this must be noted. Secondly, the cough may be *productive* or *non-productive*, depending on whether or not the person is coughing up (expectorating) sputum or, as it is more commonly called, phlegm. Although it is not pleasant, it is important to see how much phlegm is produced, and whether this is increasing or decreasing. The colour of the phlegm should also be noted – it may be yellow/green, frothy white or tinged red/pink with blood.

2. Difficulty with breathing

An elderly person with respiratory problems may, in addition to coughing, experience difficulty with breathing. This may be related to exercise. It may be noted that, after climbing stairs or walking fast, for example, the person becomes breathless. It may also be related to posture, with the patient only breathing comfortably when sitting up. In addition, the skin may be pale and the nail beds blue in colour. The person may be irritable and restless, and experience severe fatigue.

3. Observations of breathing

Other useful observations can be made of a person's breathing. The rate at which people breathe varies; certain conditions, for example a chest infection, may result in the elderly person breathing very quickly, almost gasping for air, while another condition, for example a disorder of the thyroid gland, may cause an elderly person to breathe very slowly indeed. The depth of breathing may alter, either becoming shallow, so that the chest hardly moves at all, or becoming deep, with heaving chest movements. Occasionally breathing may become irregular, the most extreme example being when breathing becomes deep and rapid, gradually tapering off until breathing stops, then gradually becoming deep and rapid again. The cycle then repeats itself and can be very frightening to watch.

Helping with breathing

1. Position

Sitting upright helps a person with breathing problems. An elderly person may be most comfortable sitting in a chair with some piece of furniture, a small table for example, with a pillow or cushion on it, placed in front, upon which he can lean. When sitting up, either in bed or in a chair, the back, neck and head should be well supported by pillows or cushions. The elderly person will probably be able to tell you which position is the most comfortable. However, it is important that he is not allowed to stay in the same position for several hours as the skin may become damaged. (This problem will be discussed in more detail in the section on pressure sores, which starts on page 83.) Movement and a change of position, even a small one, will make breathing easier and help to clear secretions from the lungs. Even a walk around the bed, or chair, every two hours can be beneficial. Anything the elderly person may need should be placed within reach – for example, tissues, a drink, reading matter and spectacles.

2. Deep breathing and coughing

Encouraging an elderly person with breathing problems to do breathing exercises regularly will be very beneficial. At the same time, the person should be encouraged to cough after every three deep breaths. If possible this should be done three or four times a day, half-an-hour or so before meals, and before retiring at night. This encourages expansion of the lungs and moves the secretions. When doing the exercises the person should be in the sitting position with hands on thighs. Make sure tissues are handy. Do not persist with the exercises if the person is obviously distressed. If he is able to expectorate phlegm it is best to allow him to rinse his mouth out with some water or a mouth wash afterwards. Allow him to rest for a while afterwards, as the exercises can be very tiring.

3. Mouth care

People with breathing problems breathe through their mouth, which becomes dry, and coughing up phlegm makes this worse and gives the mouth an unpleasant odour. It is important, therefore, that the person should be allowed to rinse his mouth with water (or a mouth wash) at regular intervals, especially after a bout of coughing and before meals. In addition, fruity drinks, ice lollies or sweets help as they stimulate the flow of saliva.

4. Fluids

Encouraging the elderly person to drink more fluids will help because the secretions in the air passages will become looser and therefore easier to cough up.

5. Cough medicines

Cough medicines are of two main types, those which prevent coughing (cough suppressants) and those which encourage coughing (expectorants). It is important that they should be given as prescribed by the doctor, and not mixed up – one cough medicine is *not* pretty much like another! Cough suppressants are prescribed for irritating non-productive coughs or when coughing is disturbing sleep. They should not be used during the day if an elderly person has excessive secretions and a productive cough. In this case they could be harmful as they would make the congestion of the lungs worse. Expectorants encourage coughing and expectoration, and are not usually given just before a person goes to bed. Finally, unless stated in the instructions, cough medicines should not be diluted with hot or cold water before they are taken.

EATING AND DRINKING
The digestive process

Food taken in through the mouth passes to the stomach and intestines and, during its passage, is changed physically and chemically. Nutrients are absorbed into the blood stream and the waste products are eliminated at the anus. In the mouth, food is chewed and mixed with saliva, making it softer and easier to swallow. The early chemical changes to some food take place in the mouth, caused by substances present in the saliva. The swallowed food passes down a tube to the stomach where it remains for about four to six hours.

The stomach is a muscular bag which contracts in a particular way to mix the food; more chemicals (enzymes) and hydrochloric acid are added until a semi-liquid consistency is achieved. In this form the semi-solid food passes into the small intestines. Further enzymes and bile are added and the final chemical changes take place. Muscular activity mixes and liquefies the food products, and the nutrients are absorbed into the blood stream. They are used by the body for the growth and repair of body tissues and to provide energy. Finally the liquid remains pass into the large intestines where, most importantly, water is absorbed from it into the blood stream. The consistency of the contents of the large intestine (now known as faeces) gradually changes from liquid to solid, in which form they are removed from the body (excreted) at the anus. This is known as the act of defaecation, or having your bowels open.

As a result of the ageing process, most elderly people retain few, if any, of their own teeth. The remaining teeth are worn down usually and the gums around them recede. The sensations of taste and smell gradually diminish with advancing age. The muscular activity of the stomach and the intestines becomes reduced and fewer fluids and chemicals are produced. The supply of blood to the intestines lessens and the absorption of nutrients from the intestines is less efficient. Abdominal muscles and the muscles at the anus weaken. All this means that the elderly person experiences loss of appetite and that food eaten is not properly digested or absorbed. Constipation often occurs and controlling defaecation is sometimes difficult. (These last two problems will be discussed on page 72.)

Assessment of eating and drinking

In the chapter on nutrition, recommended diets are discussed, but it is important to make sure that elderly people understand what their dietary needs are, and how to meet them. Also there are many factors, other than obvious illness, which may affect an elderly person's ability to take the correct diet. These include being unable to afford the best foodstuffs, problems of feeding and loss of appetite.

1. Ability to eat and drink

The most common causes of difficulty with eating and drinking are dental problems and physical handicap. Although few elderly people have their own teeth, they are reluctant, sometimes, to wear dentures or they have dentures that are ill-fitting, so that chewing is very difficult – though it is surprising how tough an elderly person's gums may be. Often, however, the gums and teeth are damaged and diseased, making eating painful and giving the mouth a bad taste, and this limits the types of food that can be eaten.

Strokes are common in elderly people and a stroke victim may be unable to use one hand and arm, which makes preparing and eating food difficult. Other conditions, such as Parkinson's disease, rheumatoid arthritis and multiple sclerosis may have the same effect.

2. Loss of appetite

Loss of appetite may occur as a result of dental problems, as described above, which may cause difficulty chewing and/or bad breath. Also the loss of the senses of taste and smell will reduce the pleasure a person gets from eating, while the slowing down of the muscular activity in the stomach increases the time food spends there. This may mean that a person is still feeling full from one meal when it is time to start eating the next. The slowness of activity in the intestines increases this effect; while constipation causes discomfort and the elderly person is, again, less inclined to eat.

3. Level of knowledge

Finally it is important to find out if the elderly person understands what foods, and how much of them, he should be taking.

Helping with eating and drinking
1. Stimulating the appetite

Whenever possible elderly people should be encouraged to have regular dental care, even those with a complete set of dentures, so that any problems can be detected early and gum disease and its associated problems treated. Ill-fitting dentures can be adjusted to provide a better fit. Having a clean mouth and being able to chew will encourage the elderly person to eat a healthier diet more easily.

The taste sensations which elderly people lose first are those of saltiness and sweetness. This means they may put excessive amounts of salt and sugar on their food. This may not be medically advisable, in which case salt and sugar substitutes should be used, large amounts of which can be taken safely. This is important as, without these flavours, food will taste bland or sour and the person will be put off eating. Taking a glass of sherry or wine before eating is also beneficial as it stimulates the appetite. However, it is important to check with the doctor first, as alcohol is not permitted when certain drugs are being taken.

Finally, if the elderly person is not preparing his own meals, food should be presented in an attractive way. It is the sight, as well as the smell, of food that stimulates the appetite. Most important of all, it is the patient's favourite food, in which he has had as much responsibility as possible in choosing and preparing, that he is most likely to enjoy eating.

2. Aids

There are a multitude of feeding devices which can be obtained (via the social services) and their use should be encouraged. These include knives, forks and spoons with special handles, gadgets to stop plates moving about, and to keep the food on the plate, and cups with shaped handles and spouts, as well as insulated plates which will keep food warmer longer. All these will encourage those who eat slowly, or who have difficulty in doing so, to try to feed themselves.

3. Position

Before old people begin to feed, or be fed, it is important that they are comfortable – they don't need to go to the toilet and they have a clean mouth. It is easiest, as most of us are aware, to eat sitting up, with food placed on a firm surface in front, where it can be seen. An elderly person who is weak or handicapped may need to be propped up with pillows or cushions in order to maintain the correct position. If the elderly person is unable to sit up, the next best thing is for him to lie on one side, with his back supported by pillows. The food can then be placed on the bed (after the sheet has been protected in some way) where it can be reached and seen. Clothes may sometimes need to be protected, but this should be done discreetly in such a way that the person does not feel humiliated – baby bibs, I would suggest, should *never* be used.

If the elderly person requires help with feeding, the helper should also be comfortable. She should be seated, facing the person. The food should be placed where it can be seen and, if the helper is right-handed, her right side should be next to the patient. When feeding, it is important to know how the person would like to receive the food, i.e. meat and vegetables separately, or all mixed up. Would he like a drink between mouthfuls, or only at the end of the meal? Do allow the person plenty of time to chew and swallow each mouthful. Don't stare at him while he is chewing; it is very disturbing, and you'll find yourself copying his chewing movements. Don't have the next mouthful hovering ready before he has finished the last. Finally, don't try to carry on a conversation throughout the meal. All these things will put the person off his meal and may stop him eating before his hunger is satisfied.

Whenever possible, encourage the person to feed himself, for example with bread and butter, biscuits, or with a drink. At the end of the meal, make sure he has a drink as this helps to rinse his mouth, and then wipe his lips clean.

4. Teaching about diet

The elderly person learns more slowly, and memory, especially for recent events, is poor. This should be taken into account when trying to teach. You should find out what the person knows already, then decide what he should learn first. There are three basic rules of teaching: first, to progress from what is known to what is unknown; second, to progress from the simple to the more complicated. (Remember, with an elderly person it may be necessary to repeat things several times, and for a few days, before important facts are remembered.) Third, praise and encouragement at regular intervals help enormously.

ELIMINATION

Fluid waste is removed (eliminated or excreted) from the body mainly through the urinary system, while solid waste is excreted through the digestive system. Problems with either of these systems can be very embarrassing and upsetting for those afflicted, and special tact and understanding are required when coping with people with such problems.

Urination

Excess water and waste substances are removed from the blood by the kidneys and combine to form urine. This urine passes down two tubes (one from each kidney) to the bladder. The bladder acts as a storage organ for the urine. When it contains about 500 ml (just under one pint), we feel the urge to urinate (pass water). If we respond, then the bladder is emptied.

As a result of the ageing process, the kidneys begin to shrivel and become less efficient at removing excess water and waste products from the blood. Therefore less urine is produced. The bladder muscles become weaker and the bladder is able to hold less urine. Also emptying the bladder becomes more difficult, and either urine dribbles out uncontrollably, or the bladder stretches and holds more urine which it cannot remove. In addition, men have a gland near the exit of the bladder (the prostate gland) which enlarges and blocks the flow of urine.

Assessment of urination

There are a variety of problems that the elderly may have with urination, which range from passing no urine at all, to passing small amounts of urine frequently. It is important, therefore, when caring for elderly patients, to make certain observations when they urinate. These observations should include the following:

1. Volume.
2. Frequency.
3. Urgency.
4. Control.
5. Difficulty/discomfort.

1. Volume

A useful way of judging how much urine is passed on each occasion is to make a comparison with a common household object. For example, a small amount (an egg cup full), a moderate amount (a mug full) and a large amount (a milk bottle full). Where it is necessary, the district nursing sister or the general practitioner will ensure that urinals/bedpans/commodes are provided for the elderly person to use at home.

2. Frequency

In addition to volume, noting how often the elderly person urinates is an important and useful observation. The simplest recording method is to ask the elderly person himself to record the time when he passes water. If he is not able to do this, those helping must take the responsibility. Complicated charts are not necessary; all that is required is a record of the time when the elderly person urinates and the volume which is passed – small, moderate or large. When an elderly person is passing small amounts of urine frequently it is distressing and tiring, as well as inconvenient. When he needs help with this activity, in addition, the experience may be many times worse for both the elderly person and the helper. However, some of the causes of this condition are simple to remedy and therefore the doctor should always be informed, in order that he may diagnose, and treat, the cause.

3. Urgency

Many elderly people are disturbed and inconvenienced, as well as sometimes embarrassed, by the fact that they get very little warning that they need to urinate. This problem will soon become apparent to those caring for the old. It is something they may be reluctant to discuss (owing to embarrassment). If elderly people are unable, sometimes, to respond fast enough and they wet themselves, they may be reluctant to leave their room, to go out, or even to have visitors.

4. Control

Incontinence occurs when a person is unable to control urination, and may even be unaware that it has occurred (as against those who are unable to respond in time). As a result, the elderly person's skin becomes soaked with urine which damages it and makes an unpleasant smell.

5. Difficulty/discomfort

An elderly person may complain of difficulty in urinating, or of a pain, or burning sensation, when urinating. When the latter occurs, the urine may be cloudy in appearance and have an unpleasant smell. Finally, it may be observed that an elderly person has passed very little, less than a mug full, of urine, or none at all, in a 24-hour period. This should be reported to a doctor promptly, as the implications may be serious.

Helping with urination

In order to help someone with problems of urination, it is useful to know, particularly, the time when they urinate and how this compares with their drinking habits. A simple chart can be designed, as shown in Table 6.

Table 6 A fluid chart

Time	Drinks	Urine
7.30		Moderate
8.00	Tea	
9.00	Tea	
10.00		Small

After a few days of such recording, it may be possible to work out the best times for taking the elderly person to the toilet, or offering a bedpan, commode or urinal. This should reduce both the problems of urgency and of incontinence. Alternatively, it may be decided that it would be better for the elderly person not to have too much to drink at a particular time of day, as nobody would be available to help him urinate. Such decisions, of course, should be made after discussion with the elderly person.

Most people prefer to go to the toilet in the privacy of the bathroom. However, if the elderly person is not able to get about very well, if he experiences urgency, or if the toilet is inaccessible, then it may be necessary to keep the utensils – urinals/bedpans/ commode – within easy reach. However, every effort should be made to keep them out of sight – for example, in a small cupboard, under the bed or in a cardboard box. A commode can be camouflaged, too. If an elderly man is using a urinal, then it is useful to put a bucket beside him. When he has used the urinal he can stand it safely in the bucket, until it can be emptied.

Apart from loss of privacy, the other unpleasant feature of using bedpans and urinals, in what is really the 'living room', is the smell. This can be controlled, however, if the utensils are emptied as soon as they are used, and then washed under running water, using a brush and a cleaning agent. In addition, an air freshener can be used.

It is possible to reduce, if not cure, incontinence in elderly people. As mentioned earlier, recording the occasions when incontinence occurs may indicate the best times to take the person to the toilet, or to offer a bedpan or urinal. Asking the elderly person at regular intervals if he needs to go to the toilet, and responding promptly if he asks to go, will also help. One effect of being incontinent is that the person is reluctant to drink anything, but this makes the problem worse. So, unless there is a medical reason against it, the elderly person should be encouraged to drink plenty – at least 4–5 pints per day. Part of the problem with incontinence is that the bladder is never emptied completely. This can, in part, be overcome in women if they are sitting upright when they urinate; with men, it is best if they stand up. With both men and women it may be necessary, if they are confused or unsteady, to stay with them while they urinate, in order to supervise and support them.

Two consequences of incontinence (that the skin is constantly soaked with urine which is damaging to it, and that the smell of urine is always present) can be reduced, to some extent, if the elderly person wears protective pads and pants. The pads soak up the urine and have a covering, like a nappy liner, which prevents most of the urine soaking the skin. It must be remembered that the pads should be changed regularly or their benefit will be lost. The protective pants keep clothing dry and, therefore, cut down on the smell. When items such as these are required, the general practitioner will normally ask the district nursing sister to visit. The district nursing sister will then order the most appropriate type of pads and pants for the elderly person to wear during the day, and make sure that he has protective sheets to put on the bed at night. She will also give advice as to the best ways to dispose of wet, disposable items.

Occasionally, it is necessary to put a tube (a catheter) into the bladder to drain out the urine. The urine then passes down into a collecting bag. In this case it is important to remember that the tubing should be inspected regularly; it should not be kinked or pinched as this will block the flow of urine. Also, the tubing and bag should be arranged so that the urine only flows downwards – draping the tubing over the arm of a chair will restrict the flow of urine. If possible, it is nicer if the bag can be placed out of sight, or covered in some way, perhaps with an old hot-water bottle cover. When a catheter is in place, the skin around it should be washed daily with warm soapy water. Finally, the district nursing sister, if she does not make daily visits, will explain how to empty the bag, and when and how to replace it.

Defaecation

Solid waste, or faeces (pronounced feecees), also called stool, is removed from the body via the rectum (the back passage). Some people defaecate (have their bowels open) each day; while, for others, the normal habit is to go only once every two or three days. However, it should be recognised that it is the habit which is normal for the individual which should be the point for assessment of changes in habit.

Assessment of defaecation

For the elderly the most common disorders of defaecation are as follows:
1. Constipation.
2. Impaction.
3. Faecal incontinence.

Other disorders, such as diarrhoea, and changes from the normal bowel habit, are caused usually by an illness, rather than by the ageing process, and should be reported to the doctor. Normal faecal matter is soft but of a firm shape, medium brown in colour and has a recognisable smell. Assessment of defaecation, therefore, should include the frequency, compared with the normal habit, the consistency of the faeces, their colour and smell. Factors other than specific diseases of the digestive system, which may alter defaecation in the elderly, include lack of exercise, poor diet, inadequate fluid intake, certain drugs and damage to the brain.

1. Constipation

As with urination, a useful way of identifying changes in the usual bowel habit is to record every bowel action on a chart. This can be done either by the elderly person or by the helper. Thus, if a person has a bowel action every day, an absence of this for a few days (two or three) means he is constipated. However, if the person usually has his bowels open less often, several more days (six or seven) must pass before it can be assumed that he is constipated.

2. Impaction

This is a more severe condition than constipation. The longer faeces are retained in the rectum, the drier and harder they become. Impaction occurs when a round, very hard lump of faeces becomes stuck in the rectum and cannot be passed. Occasionally, as a result of impaction, an elderly person may leak small amounts of liquid faecal fluid uncontrollably. The difference between this and diarrhoea is that diarrhoea is the passage of unformed (loose) stools, accompanied by a cramping pain, an urgency to defaecate, general weakness and a feeling of sickness. If it is suspected that the elderly person is suffering from faecal impaction, the doctor should be told.

3. Faecal incontinence

Some elderly people are unable to control their bowel action, for example after they have had a stroke. The faecal matter which is passed is usually of a softer consistency than normal stool, but otherwise the same.

Helping with defaecation

A few fairly simple actions, which mean only minor changes in the elderly person's way of living, may be all that is needed to solve his bowel problems, of which constipation is the most common. These actions should include exercise, increasing the amount of liquid being drunk, introducing bulk (fibre) into the diet, and ensuring a proper bowel action.

Quite a lot of useful exercise can be achieved by incorporating it into other activities, such as washing and dressing, when the elderly person should be allowed and encouraged to do as much as possible for himself. (The difficulty of this for the helper is that the tasks may take much longer to complete.) When the elderly person is moving about, he can be encouraged to take a longer route between one place and another. In addition, time may be set aside during the day as an exercise period, say 30 minutes morning and afternoon.

The importance of drinking plenty has already been mentioned, and it will help to prevent constipation. (The value of dietary fibre, and foods containing this fibre, is discussed in chapter 8.) Laxatives or other medications should only be used if increased activity, drinking more, and a high fibre diet, fail to prevent constipation, and then only on the advice of the doctor.

Finally, the elderly person should be advised and helped to go to the toilet (in the bathroom, or using a bedpan or commode) at the same time each day. If a chart has been kept of bowel actions, the best time should be easy to work out. Plenty of time should be allowed for the elderly person to defaecate, to make sure the bowel is completely emptied. If faecal incontinence is a problem, then the elderly person should go to the toilet and try to have his bowels open after every meal. As with urination, the best position for defaecation is sitting up, with the feet resting on the floor. Using a bedpan when sitting in bed is difficult, both for the elderly person and for the helper.

In conclusion, many of the problems of elimination cause elderly people discomfort and embarrassment. They restrict their social activity frequently, too, either limiting the amount they go out, or making them reluctant to invite people to visit them. Assisting an elderly person with urination and defaecation problems requires a great deal of tact on the part of the helper, not only to avoid embarrassing the elderly person further, but also to avoid humiliating him by treating him like a child. However, when these problems are cleared up, or made less severe, it is very rewarding for both patient and nurse.

WASHING, GROOMING AND DRESSING

It is generally recognised that our outward appearance is a good indication of how we are feeling and what our mood is. Usually it is safe to assume that if a person appears well groomed, with skin, hair, nails, and clothes clean and tidy, he is feeling good, while an absence of good grooming may mean that he is feeling low. However, for many elderly people, the cause of poor grooming is that they are unable, physically, to care for themselves any better; this itself makes them feel low. The effects of ageing on bones, joints, muscles and the nervous system may have an additional effect on the elderly person's ability to care adequately for himself. It is important, too, to keep our skin, nails and hair clean for a variety of health reasons.

The skin covers the body completely and should be smooth, supple, warm and unbroken. It has three main functions. Firstly, it protects the body, acting as a barrier against infection. Secondly, it helps to control our body temperature so that, for example, when we are hot, we sweat, which cools us. When we are cold, our hairs stand on end and we shiver, which helps to warm us. Thirdly, there are nerves in the skin which detect sensations, such as light and firm touch, painful touch, hot and cold temperatures, and this protects us from injury. Nails are part of the skin (in good health they are hard, smooth and rounded), and so is hair, the whole body being covered with hair except the palms of the hands and the soles of the feet. Hair is strong, not brittle, and – as can be seen best on the head – shiny. Hair grows also in the nose and ears. Two types of glands are found in the skin – those producing sweat and those producing an oily substance which keeps the skin soft and smooth and the hair shiny.

As a result of the ageing process, changes in the skin include the appearance of lines and wrinkles. The skin becomes less supple, more easily damaged, cut and scratched; and less fat is stored under the skin, so that it hangs in loose folds. Hair in the nose and ears gets thicker, while on the scalp it turns grey and thins; nails tend to become harder and brittle. There are fewer sweat glands, and those remaining do not work so well, so that less sweat is produced. The ability to detect sensations is reduced, particularly for firm touch and temperature, and sometimes for pain. In addition to the effects of ageing, the elderly person's general health, diet, and the amount of exercise he gets, affect the condition of the skin.

Elderly people's muscles lose strength, their joints get stiff, their nervous systems become impaired so that messages are not relayed to their arms and legs, and their brains get less blood so they think more slowly. All this means that an elderly person may experience difficulty carrying out simple tasks, such as washing and dressing. The effort involved may become too much for him.

Assessment of washing and grooming
The skin is constantly bathed in sweat and oil, and is covered

with small flakes of dead skin, all of which must be removed by regular washing with soap and water, otherwise the accumulations will cause unpleasant body odour and skin problems, such as infections. Areas which require special attention are the armpits, under the breasts, in the folds of the skin, and those parts affected by urine and faeces. A daily bath, however, while preferred by some people, is not essential for health.

To assess an elderly person's needs, it is necessary to know several things. How often has he been in the habit of bathing? Is he incontinent of urine and/or faeces? Are special gadgets needed to get him in and out of the bath? How much is the elderly person able to do for himself? Can he clean his own teeth? Can he wash his own hair and care for his nails? Depending on the answers to these questions, plans can be made as to the best way of keeping the elderly person clean and fresh.

Helping with washing and dressing

1. Bathing

If possible, the elderly person should be given the chance to have a tub bath once a week. A relative nursing an old person at home may need the help of a district nursing sister. It may be that the helper can manage alone if equipment, such as hoists, rails and seats, is provided by the social services. The helper should ensure the bathroom is warm and the water is the right temperature to suit the elderly person. Everything that is needed should be collected before the bath begins – soap, flannels, towels, slipmat (for the bath), nail brush and a change of clothing. The elderly person should be helped into the bath, if necessary, and then be allowed to enjoy it; he should be encouraged to wash himself as much as possible. Most people, not only the elderly, prefer to wash their own pudenda (private parts), but help may be needed to wash their back and feet. As much privacy as possible should be allowed; however, some elderly people need some supervision and this should be done as discreetly as possible.

After the bath, the patient should dry himself, or be dried, thoroughly; deodorants, creams and talcum powder should be used as he wishes. Before dressing, the skin should be inspected to see if there are any cuts or sores which require attention. Feet should be inspected to see if such conditions as corns or athlete's foot are present. Advice on their treatment may be sought from the doctor, the chiropodist or the local pharmacist.

Alternatively, if the elderly person is not having a daily bath, then a strip-wash, sitting or standing at the wash-basin, the sink or with a bowl placed on a table, is the next best thing. The routine is similar to that described above, help being given as required. The water will, of course, have to be changed regularly and a bowl will be needed for soaking the feet.

2. Washing in bed

Some elderly people are not able to cope with either bathing or having a strip-wash, in which case they will need to be washed in bed. Preparation is much the same as above; the room should be warm, privacy should be maintained and everything needed should be collected beforehand, including two bowls and two flannels. The bedclothes should be folded to the foot of the bed and the elderly person should be covered with a blanket, sheet or large towel. Any wet or soiled clothing or sheets should be removed before the wash begins. If possible, the elderly person should be sitting up, so that he can wash as much of himself as he can – face, arms and hands, chest and pudenda. If, however, the nurse has to do most of the washing and drying, the best order to follow is – face, ears, neck, chest, arms, hands, abdomen (tummy), legs, feet, back and, finally, pudenda. Wash using firm, but gentle, strokes; make sure soap is rinsed off. The water in the bowl should be as hot as the helper or nurse can stand it (it is surprising how quickly the flannel cools), and should be changed as often as necessary. The second bowl and flannel should be used for washing the buttocks (the cheeks of the bottom) and the pudenda. If flannels are sewn into a mitten shape (without the thumb), and worn on the hand, they are easier to use.

Elderly people are often very embarrassed at having what many refer to as their 'private parts' washed by another person; however, if this task is approached in a tactful, matter-of-fact way, it is usually accepted. Keeping this area clean is very important as unpleasant smells are removed and the risk of infection reduced. With women secretions collect in the folds of skin of the pudenda, and the area can become very inflamed; therefore careful cleaning is necessary. With men the area beneath the scrotum may get sweaty and inflamed; it should be cleaned very gently as the testicles are very sensitive. In uncircumcised men the foreskin needs to be retracted and the exposed area cleaned.

After the bath, the bed should be made. If the elderly person is not getting up and getting dressed, he should, if possible, sit in a chair while this goes on, as it is easier for him and the helper.

3. Care of hair

If possible, the elderly person should have his hair washed every 1–2 weeks. This is often done while he is in the bath, or it can be washed in the wash-basin/sink. (It is also possible to wash the hair of somebody confined to bed.) The elderly person's hair should be brushed and combed at least twice a day – after washing and dressing are completed, and at the end of the day. Brushing and combing short hair is not difficult, but long hair does present problems. It should be brushed and then combed, beginning at the ends and working up towards the scalp, as this is the best way to remove tangles. Elderly ladies should be asked how they would like their hair arranged; it contributes to their feeling of well-being to know their hair is done the way they would do it, if they could. The hair of elderly ladies is often so thin that holding plaits and buns in place with hair pins is very difficult.

4. Care of mouth and teeth

The daily care of mouth and teeth should be carried out using toothpaste, or other cleaning agent, and a toothbrush. If the elderly person still has any of his own teeth, these should be cleaned at least twice a day. Dentures should be removed at least once a day and cleaned under running water, using a toothbrush and a cleaning agent. When the dentures have been removed, the mouth should be cleaned – swilling round with water is usually sufficient. It is useful to remember that wet dentures are easier to put back into the mouth than dry ones. The elderly person should be encouraged to do as much as possible himself. If necessary, however, the nurse should be prepared to brush his teeth for him, brushing away from the gums in a rolling movement.

If the elderly person is confined to bed and cannot sit up, turn him on to his side. A cup of water and a straw can be used for rinsing the mouth, and a small bowl provided for spitting into. A towel should be placed under the person's head to protect the bedding and to wipe away any drips.

If decayed teeth or sore gums are noticed, they should be attended to by a dentist, as infection in the mouth can spread to the chest, making the elderly person very ill. In addition, a diet that includes food which requires chewing, and plenty to drink, encourages the flow of saliva. This helps to keep the mouth clean and fresh. Sore teeth and gums and ill-fitting dentures may mean that the elderly person is unable to eat a proper diet, and if the mouth is dirty, and has a bad taste, this will also put him off his food. Care of the mouth, therefore, is important for the elderly person's general health.

5. Shaving a man

If a man is used to being clean shaven, he will be very uncomfortable if he is unshaven. If he is unable to shave himself, then the helper must do this. However, some men, who can no longer manage a wet shave, are able to use an electric razor. Using an electric razor is certainly easier for a helper. If a wet shave is required, a thin layer of lather, made with warm water, shaving soap and a brush, is applied to the face, or shaving cream may be used. Allow a few minutes for the beard to be softened. Keep both the razor and the skin wet during the shave. Keep the skin taut with the fingers of one hand, use short strokes and shave against the direction of hair growth. Keep the razor clean by rinsing it regularly. At the end of the shave, rinse the soap off and dry the face. After a wet or an electric shave, apply aftershave lotion, if the man so wishes.

6. Dressing

The choice of clothing worn by an elderly person should be made carefully and should be suited to his personal preference. Other factors, such as any physical disability, should be taken into account. If an elderly woman is in bed and needs to use a bedpan, then a nightdress with a full-length opening at the back is the most suitable. If the elderly person is incontinent, the clothing should be of material which can withstand either being boiled or being washed in a biological washing powder.

Small buttons, hooks and eyes, zips down the back of dresses and fine nylon zips should be avoided as elderly people, who have less control over fine movements, and loss of feeling in their finger tips, find them difficult to manage. In many cases, these fasteners can be replaced, for example, with 'Velcro'. A member of the social services, usually the occupational therapist, will give advice and help in this matter. The Disabled Living Foundation's publication – Dressing for disabled people – may prove useful. It has illustrations of special garments that are available, and describes alterations which can be made to ordinary clothes. It demonstrates how people with a variety of disabilities can dress and undress themselves. It is important, when helping an elderly person with a disability to dress, that garments should be put on an affected limb first, as this is much easier. When helping an elderly person to dress himself, the helper should stand at the unaffected side, and give support if needed. It might seem more sensible to stand at the affected side, but this is not the case. The helper should support the side that helps to steady the person. When undressing, garments should be removed from the affected limb last.

Finally, body temperature tends to be lower in elderly people and they may need to wear more, and warmer, clothes than would appear to be necessary. If they are sitting in a chair, a blanket may need to be wrapped around their legs (rather than just draped over them).

The routine of washing, grooming, dressing and undressing may take quite a long time each day. It is a time when the elderly person and the helper are in close contact with each other. It can be used as an opportunity for conversation; many elderly people enjoy reminiscing, and the helper may learn a lot from the tales told. It is also a chance for the helper to keep the elderly person up to date with what is going on beyond the immediate surroundings. Most people are conscious of their appearance, and knowing they are clean and well groomed makes elderly people feel good, contributing to their sense of well-being. The care taken by the helper will reassure the elderly person of his own worth, and that he is not seen as a burden and no longer useful, even though he may not be independent.

SLEEPING
The mechanism of sleep

Sleep is a basic human need, and it is accepted that a 'good night's sleep' is necessary for mental and physical well-being, although the actual amount of sleep needed decreases as we get older. A new-born child needs about 16 hours, a teenager about $8\frac{1}{2}$ hours, and an elderly person 6 hours or less. In addition, the amount of time spent in really deep sleep diminishes as we get older. Therefore, because an elderly person does not sleep as soundly, his sleep may be disturbed by things which would not affect a younger person.

Assessment of sleeping

It is important to remember when considering how elderly people are sleeping, to discuss the matter with them. Your idea of how well, or how badly, they are sleeping may not agree with theirs. Their views should always be considered when planning and preparing them for sleep. Factors which disturb an elderly person's sleep may include: a troublesome cough, breathing difficulties, hunger, going to the toilet, and pain.

Helping with sleep

A major factor in helping the elderly to sleep well is to make sure they are comfortable. In addition, they should be tired and ready to sleep when they go, or are put, to bed. It is important to remember that an elderly person, while requiring less sleep, probably needs more rest than a younger person. Therefore the day's activities should be planned to include periods of rest, but not sleep, as 'cat-naps' during the day are a major cause of sleeping difficulty. The elderly person should be encouraged to do something which keeps him mentally alert while allowing physical rest, for example playing cards, doing a jigsaw puzzle, or something similar.

1. Cough

If the elderly person has a troublesome cough this should be dealt with as described earlier. When preparing an elderly person for sleep it is important to ensure that his chest is clear, and then he should take a linctus. This clearing of the chest will also help the person with breathing difficulties. It is also important to accept that many elderly people are more comfortable if they sleep sitting in a chair, rather than lying in bed.

2. Hunger

Many elderly people do not feel like having, or are not able to have, two or three meals a day. For them, and for others, a warm milky drink and a biscuit or a small snack for the last meal of the day will help to make them more comfortable for sleeping.

3. Toileting

One of the last things elderly people should be encouraged to do, before settling down for the night, is to go to the toilet. Following this, toilet facilities should be readily available and accessible during the night. If they can get to the bathroom, then the way should be clear of any obstacles, and a light should be left on in the bedroom and in the bathroom. Otherwise, a commode, bedpan, or urinal should be placed close to the bed, and again a light should be left on in the bedroom.

4. Pain

Because an elderly person does not sleep very soundly many discomforts may disturb his sleep. These may include aching joints, night cramps, an uncomfortable bed, and feeling cold. To relieve these problems, one of the first things to do is to make sure that the mattress isn't lumpy, and that it provides a firm support. A lumpy, sagging mattress will cause many aches and pains. When making the bed, the most important thing to do is to make sure it will be comfortable for the user. To achieve this, the undersheet should be tight and smooth, and the top sheet and blankets should be large enough to tuck in all round, whilst leaving room for the occupant to move around freely. Tight upper bedclothes will force the feet into a cramped position. There should be enough bedclothes to keep the person warm, but these should not be so heavy as to be uncomfortable. If practical, a 'fleecy' underblanket is very good; and many elderly people prefer a duvet for the warmth it gives without the extra weight. Warming the bed before use will also be helpful. If a hot-water bottle is used, it should be removed before the elderly person gets into bed. Electric underblankets should be switched off before the bed is occupied. If necessary, extra pillows or cushions should be used to support joints and limbs.

If the elderly person has a lot of pain, then, after discussion with the general practitioner or the district nursing sister, pain-relieving tablets may be given. The best time to give them is before the person is prepared for bed, as then they will be starting to work once they are in bed.

Elderly people often have difficulty getting to sleep once they are in bed. Watching television, listening to the radio, reading or being read to, as preferred, may help them to relax and settle down to sleep. Only as a last resort should sedatives (medicines which make you sleep) be used, as they often make elderly people sleep deeper and longer than they need to. They wake up with chest congestion and stiff joints. The drugs also lower the body temperature, which is not a good thing, and, because of the way they work, elderly people wake up groggy and confused.

If the measures described here are carried out and elderly people are comfortable and relaxed when they are in bed, then they are more likely to sleep well. Finally, as mentioned earlier, it must be remembered that elderly people need less sleep than younger people. If they are put to bed early, say at eight or nine o'clock, then they cannot be expected to sleep until seven or eight o'clock in the morning. When planning the time an elderly person goes to bed at night and rises in the morning, his needs should be considered first.

In a study conducted in 1977, it was estimated that the cost to the National Health Service (NHS) of treating pressure sores was in the region of £60 million. It must have risen considerably since then. However, most, if not all, pressure sores are preventable; and the cost of prevention is much less than the cost of treatment – to the potential victims and to the NHS.

The mechanism of pressure sore development

The skin, with the exception of the outer layer, is living tissue, so it needs a constant supply of blood. This is provided by a network of very fine blood vessels which gives the skin its pink colour, supplies it with oxygen and nourishment, and removes waste products from it. If pressure is applied to the skin, then these fine blood vessels will be squashed and the flow of blood stopped. The area affected will not receive the necessary supply of oxygen and nutrients, and the waste products will not be removed.

The skin can tolerate a lot of pressure for a short time; but a little pressure for a long time will disrupt the blood supply. If you hold an empty glass in your hand, you can see how even a small amount of pressure will make the parts of your hand touching the glass go white. The blood supply to these surfaces has been cut off. The most common sites for pressure sores to develop are where points of bone are found close to the surface of the skin. When pressure, usually in the form of body weight, is applied to these areas, the tissues between bone and skin surface are compressed. If pressure continues, the blood flow is interrupted, with the effect that, after 30 minutes, tissue damage occurs. However these effects are reversible if pressure does not continue for more than two hours. This damage occurs because the tissue is deprived of oxygen and nourishment, and waste products accumulate. This results in localised swelling, which in turn increases the pressure on the tissues and fine blood vessels. If pressure is unrelieved, the tissue dies, and this is how a pressure sore is caused.

Pressure sore development has four main stages, as follows:
1. Pressure causes redness of the skin without tissue damage. Shortly after pressure is relieved, the redness disappears.
2. Prolonged pressure causes slight damage to fine blood vessels and local tissue. First, there is congestion. If an area of red skin is pressed continuously, it remains red (healthy skin would go white when pressed, then go red again when the pressure was removed). Second, blistering occurs.
3. If pressure continues, the deeper layers of the skin are damaged, the blister breaks down and an ulcer (pressure sore) appears. (Friction as well as, or in addition to, pressure will cause a pressure sore. An everyday example of this is the damage caused by new shoes which are too tight.)
4. Finally, the ulcer becomes infected, gangrene may be present and, occasionally, the underlying bone becomes infected, too.

Assessment of risk

Many of the features of the ageing process increase the elderly person's chance of developing a pressure sore. Poor functioning of the heart and lungs means less oxygen going to the tissues; while slowing down of the digestive system means less nourishment is available. Elderly people are less active, take less exercise, and immobility increases the risk of pressure sore development. In addition, there is loss of feeling, especially for pressure and pain. Their skin tends to be dry and fragile, which makes it more easy to damage, and it heals more slowly. Finally, many of the diseases to which the elderly are susceptible increase the risk, for example, of heart disease and stroke. Assessment must include consideration of the elderly person's physical and mental state. The assessment should include the following factors:
1. Physical condition.
2. Mental condition.
3. Activity.
4. Mobility.
5. Incontinence.

1. Physical condition

Some elderly people are well nourished, have soft, supple skin, with normal feeling, and no major illness. Others are either too fat or too thin, they are undernourished and have dry, fragile skin. They have some loss of feeling and often have one or more serious illness. Those in the second group are very likely to develop pressure sores.

2. Mental condition

Although elderly people's mental processes may be slower than they used to be, they may still be very alert. It may be evident, from questioning them, or from listening to their conversation, that they know where they are and that they recognise the people they meet. In addition they can recite the date, and know what the time is and what day of the week it is. They are also as interested in local and national events as they used to be. Others, however, have no interest in what is going on around them; they may be very confused as to time, place and events. Finally, there are those who appear to be permanently half asleep. The less alert and the more confused an elderly person is, the greater his risk of getting pressure sores.

3. Activity

An elderly person's level of activity may range from being able to walk around unaided, to being able to walk only with the help of another person. He may be able to get from bed to chair and back with help but, once in the chair, he cannot get up, or he may have to remain in bed all the time. The less active the elderly person is, the more he is at risk.

4. Mobility

An elderly person may have good use and movement of all limbs and joints, or, at the other end of the scale, he may be unable to move himself at all. The less mobile a person is, the more he is at risk.

5. Incontinence

Some elderly people have complete control over their urination and defaecation, while, at the other extreme, there are those who are incontinent of urine and faeces. Other elderly people may be incontinent occasionally, or incontinent of only urine, or of only faeces. Those who are incontinent are at risk, and those doubly incontinent are most at risk.

Each of these five factors must be taken into account when assessing elderly people for risk of developing pressure sores. The aim of care must be to improve their condition, in all the areas where they are at risk, by improving their performance, or by reducing the risk to the minimum. A doctor writing in a medical journal several years ago said: 'Skilled nursing care is generally accepted to be effective in preventing pressure sores.' The nursing care required may be given by anybody who finds herself caring for an elderly person.

Prevention of pressure sores

The most important single factor in preventing pressure sores is the regular, frequent change of the elderly person's position – at least every two hours. Whenever possible, the patient should be encouraged to move himself, as the actual activity is also beneficial. Quite small changes which alter slightly the area taking the weight are useful. If the elderly person is sitting in a chair, then standing up, or being stood up, each time will help. If the elderly person is in bed, his position can be altered from lying on his back to lying on one side or the other. The changes of position should be organised so that he is lying on his side for meals. However, whenever an elderly person is being moved, care must be taken to ensure that he is lifted clear of whatever he is resting on; he should not be dragged or pulled, as this may cause damage by friction. Care should be taken to ensure that sheets and clothing are free of rucks and creases.

There are a variety of pressure-relieving aids available, including pillows, sheepskins and alternating pressure mattresses and pillows. These may be used to protect bony areas that are more exposed to pressure. Pillows may be used for heels, ankles and elbows; sheepskins for the back and shoulders; alternating pressure mattress for the whole body; and pillows for the bottom, when sitting up. However, it should be remembered that these are aids to, and not substitutes for, other care being given. They help to reduce pressure on people who are particularly at risk, but regular change of position is still necessary. Creams should be applied to the skin if they are recommended by the doctor and, if they are used, they should be applied gently, not rubbed in vigorously. Before each application the skin should be thoroughly cleaned and dried, removing the previous layer of cream. Rubbing and massaging bony areas of skin should *never* be carried out as this does not improve the circulation, and it may cause further damage.

Finally, if any area of skin becomes discoloured, pressure on it should be avoided until it returns to normal. Areas of broken skin should be covered with an Elastoplast dressing, which should be replaced daily, or when it becomes wet. Again pressure should be avoided until these heal. If the discolouration or broken skin does not improve within a couple of days, the doctor should be notified.

Additional, supportive care should include ensuring that the elderly person is receiving a nourishing, well-balanced diet with plenty to drink, that he is exercising as much as possible, and that areas of skin affected by sweat, urine and faeces are washed frequently and dried thoroughly.

Pressure sores are painful and unpleasant; they take much longer to heal in the elderly. They are harmful to an elderly person's general health and costly to the NHS. This is surely a case where 'an ounce of prevention is worth a pound of cure'.

Further reading

Roper, N., Logan, W. W., Tierney, A. J., *The Elements of Nursing* (Churchill Livingstone, 1980).

6

MAINTAINING A SAFE ENVIRONMENT

RUTH MANLEY

formerly Professional Adviser,
Society of Geriatric Nursing,
Royal College of Nursing

Wherever an old person is being nursed, care must be exercised to provide not only comfortable, but also safe, surroundings. But in this lies a danger of being over-protective and of depriving him of his independence. However, it is possible, with reasonable foresight, to ensure safety and security for older people which increases their ability to move about their home, their room, or the hospital ward, with greater confidence.

Faced with the loss of mobility, poor eyesight or hearing, older people cannot react as quickly to a stumble or trip as younger people, nor are they able to recognize a potential hazard in time to avoid it. Whether they are cared for at home, in hospital, residential home or nursing home, prevention (of accidents) should be a key word for those who look after them.

Floors and stairs, or steps, are major accident black spots. Obstacles, including pets or trailing flexes, are seldom seen before they are encountered; even a crawling baby can be a potential stumbling-block. It should be a firm rule that floors are kept clear at all times, with low pieces of furniture, such as stools, kept out of the main thoroughfare. Slip mats are much beloved by some old people, but they may be persuaded to give them up if the dangers are spelt out.

Ward floors and corridors in hospitals or homes are often shiny and reflect light, giving an impression of water; this causes patients or residents to take unnecessary avoiding action, leading to loss of balance and a fall. Adjustment of lighting can eliminate this effect. Worn, frayed carpets, particularly on stairs, are very dangerous; even the low heel of a flat shoe can catch and project the person forward with considerable force, which increases the damage on impact. If the carpet cannot be renewed, or securely fastened down, its removal may be the only remedy.

Trying to support one's weight on an unstable piece of furniture often results in a fall, usually with the weight of the fitting on top of one. Nurses must warn patients as often as is necessary of the danger of using bedside lockers as 'hoists' when trying to stand. Many are on wheels, and the wardrobe type are too light to offer support to heavy people. The wheels of hospital beds must always be kept locked, otherwise they, too, will slip away as the patient balances on the edge. In the home it may be possible to select a room with a fitted wardrobe or solid heavy furniture which is very stable, and castors or wheels can be removed from beds or divans, although some adjustment may be required to restore the height.

FINANCE

Elderly people are among the poorest in society, but some are poorer than they should be. A combination of fierce independence, and failure to claim benefit to which they are entitled, or to spend savings set aside for a rainy day, is the result of a thrifty upbringing. We can help by being alert for signs of financial hardship, whatever the cause. Inadequate heating and clothing can lead to hypothermia, and a poor diet may seriously affect health. We must persuade elderly people that independence, cherished so dearly, may depend on remaining fit and active and that money spent in order to achieve this is well spent.

Heating and lighting

Older people have a mistaken belief that they cannot afford to spend money on home repairs or maintenance; every effort should be made to persuade them to enter their retirement with a home in good decorative and structural state. Adequate heating – to prevent hypothermia – and good lighting – to minimise accidents – are essential features of a safe home for someone who is old. Financial embarrassment can prevent an even temperature being maintained in very cold weather. This is especially important for people who may not feel cold even when the body temperature is very low.

Electrical wiring and fittings in old houses can cause fire, and plugs that are not at a convenient height may result in accidents.

The Electricity Board should be asked to check wiring which is suspected of failing to reach an acceptable standard of safety.

Elderly people should be observed to see how they manage in the kitchen. Their ability to manage taps and switches, and the degree of manual dexterity with which pots and pans are handled, should be noted particularly. Modifications, without major alteration to, or replacement of, equipment can be made to overcome loss of skill caused by stiff fingers or joints. Forgetfulness with matches or gas taps is a cause of concern to neighbours, who fear the risk of fire or explosion.

All heating systems and heaters need to be thoroughly overhauled and serviced, to render them safe, efficient, and less wasteful, in order to reduce bills. Someone who has diminished sensation in hands or feet is at risk from fires or heaters which are not properly and safely guarded. It is important, therefore, to check that guards meet safety guidelines.

Fear of high electricity bills sometimes leads to the use of low voltage bulbs that give insufficient light for someone getting up at night to go to the toilet, placing him at risk from a fall, or exposure, if he is unable to get back to bed. Poor lighting, or lights which create shadows, can be overcome by replacing heavy net or lace curtains with lighter fabric, or by altering the position of overhead or wall fittings. Strip lighting is most effective in reducing shadows, if it can be provided.

Diet

Elderly people are sometimes reluctant to spend money on their food, too. An inadequate diet, which is lacking in nutrients and vitamins, leads to tiredness or deficiency disease, especially in someone who is unable to absorb essential vitamins or elements. Fresh fruit and vegetables provide most of the Vitamin C necessary to good health, and is likely to be excluded from the diet in winter when supplies are scarce and expensive. Alternative sources of supply are found in fruit juices or in ascorbic acid tablets. (This is discussed in detail in chapter 8.)

Someone living alone may be offered meals on wheels to replace the midday meal. These meals do not always meet the preference of the old person concerned, making it necessary for a regular assessment of the amount being consumed to be made. Meals for elderly people have to offer visual appeal, as well as flavour, because appetite, sense of smell and taste diminish with age.

Security

A telephone bestows a sense of security to those who live alone, providing a life-line in an emergency, and enabling relatives to keep in regular touch. The cost may be a deterrent, especially if a telephone has to be installed, but the outlay is justified if it enables independent living at home, instead of residential care. Some local authorities, and other agencies, have set up a service which contacts disabled people who live alone every day, in order to check on their well-being. Volunteers are given a small number of dependent people to look after, and expenses toward the cost of the telephone calls. The service provides help in an emergency and ensures that someone at risk is contacted each day. No reply alerts the volunteer of the need to investigate. Such a service could be usefully expanded by reducing elderly people's isolation and encouraging their verbal skills.

Different values

To achieve any change in the physical living conditions of someone who is elderly, possibly disabled, and has problems with communication requires tact, humour, the ability to listen and understand, as well as infinite patience. Values in each generation are different; facilities we take for granted may not be considered necessary by our elders, so that we have to exercise caution when proposing sweeping changes in the face of opposition. Risk, as we perceive it, may not be similarly recognised by someone who has lived out his life in such conditions. The desire to prolong life is likely to be less important than maintaining the status quo in the home environment, and should be respected as far as possible. It is often anxious relatives or neighbours who are most enthusiastic about ensuring safety.

THE ENVIRONMENT

If the patient is being nursed at home, you must first decide which is the most suitable room for him. It should be near the bathroom and toilet, and on the same level. (A local authority home improvement grant may be available in order that a downstairs cloakroom could be added, or doorways could be modified to give access to a wheelchair.) It should not be too quiet or isolated from the rest of the family, or the patient will be lonely. It should be well lit and heated, airy, clean, cheerful and bright, and not draughty. It should not be too small, and there should be plenty of room on both sides of the bed, to make nursing easier. It should not be too near the stairs, which should be guarded.

Most people are attached to their own bed and, unless there is a very strong reason for a special type of bed, they will be happier to keep their own. It is possible to hire or borrow special mattresses through the District Nursing Service or Social Services departments, or the Red Cross, if they are needed. A single bed with tables on both sides helps to keep most necessities near at hand, such as radio, spectacles, books or tissues, as well as a clock and a drink. A bedside lamp and a handbell are also useful.

A variable-height table which can be placed over the bed is useful for meals, especially breakfast, or a late-night drink. It is, however, important that old people are encouraged to get up as much as possible, to dress in ordinary day clothes, and keep normal hours. Otherwise pressure sores, contractures, renal stasis, and other ills, quickly follow.

Hospital staff, and staff in residential or nursing homes, have to be aware of the importance of mobility and rest. Getting someone out of bed and into a chair is not mobilisation, it only changes the patient's position. All old people being cared for in hospitals or homes should be offered the opportunity to rest on their beds following the midday meal. This aids digestion, and renal function, prevents swelling of the legs and feet (oedema), and, most of all, increases comfort and helps to maintain joint mobility.

For someone who is incontinent, or who is unable to reach the toilet, a commode is essential. How this is arranged or managed requires a great deal of thought and some experiment. To preserve dignity and privacy at the same time is of paramount importance; it may be possible to arrange furniture so that the commode is screened from immediate observation by someone entering the room. The problem of emptying, and the control of odour, are also vital considerations, and much trial and error will be needed before the right solution is reached. In hospital there are alternative methods of helping patients with their excretory needs, but staff need to be specially vigilant about the privacy and dignity of their patients, which may be forgotten in the hurly burly of a busy ward.

Hospitals are places for sick people but it is possible, with thought, to create a welcoming and friendly atmosphere by allowing the patient to have a few personal belongings around him, such as photographs, ornaments or other favourite possessions. The old person's room at home needs to be kept as domestic as possible, and a tendency to turn it into a mini-hospital should be fiercely resisted.

The noise level in a hospital ward can be a source of discomfort and annoyance to elderly patients. It is usually well above the noise level at home, owing to nurses talking and using equipment. It is important to remember to modulate your voice, wear quiet shoes, handle equipment quietly, and not to bang doors. It is also necessary to control the volume of radio and television in day rooms and wards, or public rooms in residential homes. Noise may also be a problem at home where space is restricted.

Medicines

One of the nurse's most important tasks is to see that the patient takes his medication in the right dosage, at the right time and in the right way, and to observe him carefully for adverse side-effects. As Dr Josephs pointed out in chapter 4, many elderly patients suffer from several different conditions at the same time, each one requiring treatment. The risk here is that the different drugs given for each condition may interact with each other, causing further problems, such as gastric upsets, wheezing, confusion, etc. The nurse must be particularly vigilant in watching for problems of this kind and in reporting them quickly.

Dr Josephs has also mentioned the problem of poor compliance with elderly patients, who may get confused about the pills they have to take, and forget whether they have taken them or not. Here, too, the nurse has the important task of overcoming this problem, and ensuring that no mistakes are made with medication. She must also make sure that all medicines are kept safely, and must keep a careful check on the quantities taken, recording them on the patient's notes. It is very important that elderly patients should only take those drugs specifically prescribed for them as individuals. In hospitals there are routines for safe drug administration, but in the home there is not the same supervision and double-checking by nurses, so all the more care is needed.

EMOTIONAL SECURITY

A sick elderly person has particular emotional needs, whether at home or in hospital. He is at his most vulnerable, he may be afraid of the future, in pain or discomfort. If in hospital, he will be feeling lonely and bereft, and will need as much warmth, reassurance and comfort as he can get. By the tone of voice, a smile, by a gentle touch, or even a hug, a good nurse will give patients this comfort and reassurance, making them feel they are still important and recognised as individuals. However, not everyone likes to be touched by comparative strangers, and some may regard this as unwelcome and over-familiar behaviour, so great tact has to be used in making the first approach.

Spiritual needs must not be forgotten. The older generation are more likely to hold religious beliefs than young people today, and are used to attending church regularly. They are also more likely to return again to their religious faith late in life, if they had abandoned it in their youth. Here again, great tact and discretion must be used in finding out the patients' beliefs, and enabling them to get the spiritual comfort they need.

Many old people possess pets, and it has been scientifically proved that they benefit greatly, both mentally and physically, from pet ownership. During a period of illness the companionship of a beloved cat, dog, or bird can give enormous comfort, but all too often this is the time when owner and pet are separated. At home, the sick elderly should be encouraged to have the company of their pets, and, even in hospital, pets should be brought to visit their owners if at all possible, as this will relieve their minds that the animal is being well cared for and has not forgotten its owner.

Perhaps the most distressing feature of being old is loneliness, and it is one which is most difficult for anyone caring for elderly people to overcome. In a busy hospital, ward staff may have little time to spend with individual patients, making it necessary for every contact to be meaningful, providing an opportunity to talk to the person, rather than, as sometimes happens, just issue instructions or give physical care. Even at home with a loving family, isolation can occur. Everyone has their own interests and lives to lead, and caring is sometimes seen in terms of meeting physical needs, forgetting that recreation and social contact are equally important to the quality of life.

A safe environment is more than just preventing accidents, or keeping someone clean, adequately nourished, and warm. A feeling of safety and security stems from confidence that people around elderly folk accept them, and accept that they have a contribution to make, no matter how small, to the family or community in which they live.

THE CONFUSED OLD PERSON

The safety of someone who is confused, disorientated, or has lost the ability to discriminate, poses a special challenge to nurses. Hyperactivity and wandering is difficult to accommodate in a busy hospital ward, and often leads to physical restraint in an effort to reduce the risk of the patient wandering away into possible danger. A demented old person's desire to wander from the safety of the house or garden has to be weighed carefully against the degree of personal harm which may result. Security becomes restrictive for such a person and is not understood or welcomed by someone who has lost the ability to discriminate. Some methods of restraint are unacceptable. For example, no patient should be forcibly confined to a bed or chair in such a way as to prevent adequate movement, by using cot-sides, or a chair which they cannot get out of. Indeed, the risk of injury is often increased by the inappropriate use of restraining chairs or rails. A really active and determined person will manage to get out, even if the chair is overturned, or he falls out of bed in the process.

Effort is better used in attempting to redirect the patient's attention by diversional activity, by physical exercise, or by providing space where they may wander safely. Tiring them out is a better management technique than tying them down. Such an approach requires team effort, so that all members of staff co-operate in providing care, and ensure relief for each other.

At home, there may be no help available; community staff must monitor the effect on the spouse, or other relative, of supporting an elderly confused person at home. Relief at regular intervals, which is reliable, is essential if home care is to continue. Additional help is necessary at other times, such as a wedding, a funeral, or other family events, or in times of sickness; even a common cold can lower resistance and tolerance levels very substantially. Volunteers or neighbours who are willing to offer an occasional 'sitting' service are invaluable aides not only to safety but also to sanity.

Wherever possible, the largest area should be made safe. Ward doors can have special closing mechanisms which require co-ordination of hand, eye, and understanding to open them. Psychiatric hospitals and their grounds offer large areas in which patients can wander with reasonable safety. However institutional care should be regarded as a last resort.

All newly designed units for the elderly should incorporate a 'safe' area where patients or residents can move at will, and come to no harm. At home it is possible to give some space for movement, provided that the problem of incontinence is being satisfactorily managed. Access to a garden is of enormous benefit.

CONCLUSION

As we have seen, as we grow older our world contracts. Home, previously a refuge, may prove hazardous when physical and mental ability declines. Reasonably fit and active people can compensate for inadequacies and inconveniences in the environment, but this ability decreases with age, especially when associated with illness or sensory loss. Immobility, or incontinence, can be induced by unsuitable accommodation, distance from the toilet, or accidental injury resulting from a fall, precipitated by poor property maintenance, and, as a result, independence may be lost, leading to residential care if support at home cannot be offered. Such a step threatens the security of someone whose home provides the only link with normality, and depression or withdrawal results. Illness, increasing infirmity and reduced mobility endanger independence, and the immediate objective must be to adapt the home to meet the new circumstances. It is hoped that this chapter has provided useful advice, for both relatives and nursing staff, to enable elderly people to be cared for in a safe environment.

7

HELPING WITH COMMUNICATION

RUTH MANLEY

formerly Professional Adviser,
Society of Geriatric Nursing,
Royal College of Nursing

We take the ability to communicate so much for granted that it is not until we lose temporarily our power of speech, hearing or sight, through illness or accident, that we become aware of the isolation suffered by those who are permanently unable to communicate. All members of the animal kingdom communicate with each other. Some, such as whales and dolphins, have been the subject of scientific studies. None, however, has developed such sophisticated methods of communication as humans, nor do they appear to suffer the same degree of isolation when communication with others breaks down.

COMPONENTS OF COMMUNICATION

In order for a person to communicate effectively, the necessary organs, nerves and muscles have to be co-ordinated. In addition, the speaker needs to have the ability to think and to express thoughts in language which has meaning for both him and the listener. The communicator has the responsibility for ensuring that his message is understood by the person he is addressing, and must remember not to use technical words, or nursing jargon, when talking to a patient. Simple language and familiar words should be used when talking to someone who is hard of hearing or confused.

We have five sensory organs – the eyes, the ears, the nose, the skin and the tongue – which together tell us about our environment. Two senses – hearing and speech – are essential to verbal communication, while sight and touch are equally important for someone who is deaf. Unfortunately we suffer a diminution of visual acuity (sharpness of outline) as a result of ageing; our eyes become presbyopic (affected by old age), and corrective lenses are prescribed to restore vision. Presbycusis, or hearing loss associated with old age, causes us to accuse people of mumbling.

Food may taste less appetising because the sense of smell is diminished and no longer stimulates appetite. Sense of touch may be impaired as a result of nerve or circulatory failure. Luckily, for most people sensory loss is very slow and does not affect all the organs at the same time nor to the same degree, so that they are able to adjust to the new circumstances. However, when sudden illness or an accident results in immediate loss, such as aphasia (disturbance or loss of the ability to comprehend or express speech) following a cerebro-vascular accident (CVA), the communication difficulties may at first appear over-whelming.

Sudden illness may result in admission to hospital and this is a frightening experience for most of us. The environment is unfamiliar and we do not know the layout of the ward or where the toilet is, or how we are expected to behave toward the staff or other patients. For an elderly patient with impaired vision, hearing or speech, admission is far more threatening and extra time is necessary to help him to settle down. Someone who is partially sighted, or blind, deaf, or confused, is at risk of misinterpreting the words and actions of those who are trying to provide care, so nurses must learn how to give information, reassurance and sympathy, clearly and simply.

HELPING WITH ADMISSION

Greeting a patient by name indicates that he is expected and welcome and also provides the opportunity for the nurse to note the patient's level of response and whether there is an obvious loss of hearing or speech. A long journey or wait before reaching the ward may make a visit to the toilet the patient's first priority; the nurse who anticipates and fulfils this need will reduce anxiety and create confidence which is essential to understanding. The patient should be introduced to the occupants of adjacent beds and then left to undress and unpack, if capable of doing so; a relative or friend will be happy to assist if encouraged to do so.

A tendency to go through the admission procedure quickly – cramming information about the ward layout, visiting times, meals, clothing, and collection of the pension book, into a few minutes – must be resisted firmly by the admitting nurse, as patients cannot absorb too many new ideas at once, and their anxiety affects their ability to express feelings. Only information which is vital to immediate care should be given at the time of admission, and the accompanying relative or friend should be present when the nursing history is noted down unless the patient is obviously unwilling for them to be present.

When noting down an elderly patient's history, or talking to someone with communication problems, it is important to observe the following rules:

1. Sit directly opposite the patient in a relaxed and attentive manner.
2. Adjust the lighting so that the speaker and the listener can see each other clearly, without light shining into the patient's eyes.
3. Make sure that the patient's glasses or hearing aid are worn, and note whether they are being used correctly.
4. Speak clearly.
5. Use language which can be understood by the patient – simplicity is the keynote.
6. Use short sentences and be brief.
7. Allow sufficient time for the patient to frame an answer and to articulate it.
8. Ask general questions first which give the patient the opportunity to demonstrate voice quality, hearing level, sight, and the state of the mouth (particularly if dentures are ill fitting and affect the quality of speech).

HEARING

The ear is divided into three parts: the external and middle ear are concerned with the collection and conduction of sound waves, and the internal ear acts as the reception area. The auditory nerve provides the pathway along which the impulses are transmitted to the interpretative centres in the brain.

Deafness

When hearing loss is complete, the risk factor is very high, for not only is the ability to communicate with others severely affected, but also the person may remain in ignorance of impending disaster until too late. A deaf person cannot hear an approaching car, or fire alarm bells, so the delay between an early warning and visual observation may be fatal.

Hearing loss is a common feature of ageing, sometimes due to a simple reversible cause, such as an accumulation of cerumen (wax) in the auditory canal. This can be removed quickly by the doctor or nurse by syringe or by using special drops to dissolve the wax.

Upper respiratory tract infection leading to blockage of the Eustachian tubes, or a middle ear infection, are other causes of temporary loss of hearing, but these may lead to permanent loss if left untreated. Any hearing loss of short duration, or persistent noises in the ears, should be investigated in order that treatment can be given.

Conductive deafness is common in old age because sound waves are not transmitted to the internal ear by the tiny bones (ossicles) of the middle ear, and do not reach the auditory nerve for transmission to the brain. Disease or disturbance of the external or middle ear, or the oval window, such as calcification of the ossicles, or chronic ear infection, are likely causes. In perceptive deafness, the disorder lies in the auditory nerve, or the auditory centre of the brain, which means that the sound impulses cannot be interpreted.

The following are rules for speaking to someone who is 'hard of hearing':

1. Make sure the person is attending.
2. Speak toward the 'best' ear.
3. Ensure that the patient can see your face and lips.
4. Do not exaggerate lip movements.
5. Speak normally and clearly.
6. Use short sentences and repeat if necessary.
7. Be patient and do not overtire the person.
8. Do not sit too close to the patient with a hearing aid – about 1½ metres is near enough.

When hearing has been totally lost do the following:

1. Use written messages, slates, picture cards, symbols, or sign language, if speech is also affected.
2. Encourage patients to speak at every opportunity in order that they maintain the function of the muscles of their lips, mouth and throat.

Menière's syndrome

This disorder of the internal ear causes progressive hearing loss and is particularly distressing for the patient because of the nausea, vomiting, tinnitus (singing noises) and severe vertigo which accompany the episodes. Patients should be nursed quietly in bed during the attack and may require cot-sides to ensure their safety if vertigo is a marked feature. Other patients may need to be reassured that not all noises in the ears lead to Menière's syndrome.

SIGHT

The eyeball contains specialised cells – the retina – which are sensitive to light rays focused through the refractive media of the eye, in a similar way to a camera, the image being interpreted by the visual centre of the brain. Loss of sight threatens our ability to move about freely and safely, or to orientate to new situations as quickly as sighted people. Someone who has lost his sight has also lost the stimulation of change of scenery, of travelling, or the enjoyment of theatre, ballet and television. Patients who suffer accidental injury to their eyes are naturally fearful and anxious about the effect of reduced vision on their physical, psychological, social and emotional well-being. Older people also worry about their ability to remain in their own homes; rehabilitation for irreversible blindness is more difficult in late life.

Blindness leads to loss of the visual contact with others which forms a vital part of normal social exchange. The eye conditions associated with ageing tend to develop slowly, requiring regular ophthalmic examination, and change of lenses to correct the refractive errors that cause the light rays to be deflected from the retina. Many systemic disorders, such as diabetes mellitus or hypertension, produce exudates or haemorrhages in the retinal blood vessels which lead to retinopathy if untreated. Someone complaining of reduced vision should be examined medically to exclude underlying disorders.

Presbyopia (old sight) is the result of diminished visual acuity which starts in the middle years of life and is compensated for by the use of glasses, especially for reading or close work. In later years, both distance and near vision may require assistance, and bifocal lenses are prescribed, creating problems for some old people when using steps or stairs.

Cataract, or opacity of the lens of the eye, is a common condition of later life, causing increasing loss of vision in people over the age of 50. When there is a marked loss of sight, the opaque lens is removed surgically, an operation with a high success rate. Following its removal, the patient requires new glasses with an extra lens to replace the one removed.

Glaucoma, an eye condition in which the internal pressure of the eye is raised, causing pain and loss of sight, is less responsive to treatment than cataract, but relief can be gained from a combination of drugs or surgical drainage. If left untreated, glaucoma causes permanent optic nerve damage, leading to blindness.

The following are rules for helping someone with impaired vision:

1. Reduce his anxiety by providing the opportunity to talk.
2. Orientate him carefully with his new environment.
3. Explain the layout of the premises and allow a mobile patient to explore them.
4. Always speak to the patient before approaching too closely.
5. Always address him by name, so that he knows you are speaking to him.
6. Always tell the patient you are leaving the room or vicinity.
7. Check that the environment is safe, in order to prevent accidents.
8. Answer all questions and ensure understanding.
9. Encourage participation in ward activity.
10. Seek stimulation and activities for the patient which prevent boredom and provoke interest.
11. Use books, the radio and tape recorders, in order to stimulate conversation.

SPEECH

Vocal sound is produced in the larynx by the vocal cords. The larynx is part of the respiratory tract, lying at the root of the tongue, below the oro-pharynx and above the trachea. The vocal cords are two folds of thick mucous membrane that lie at each side of the larynx (see Fig. 5).

When the cords are relaxed, the passage of air through them makes no sound, but when they are contracted, the cords shorten, coming close together in the centre of the larynx (see Fig. 6). Sound is produced as the cords vibrate when air is squeezed through them, the force of the contraction giving pitch to the voice. All the respiratory organs are involved in the production of sound, but the larynx and the vocal folds are specially concerned; the speech centre and the nerves controlling the movement of the tongue and jaw are of special importance. The size of the larynx varies, and is one reason for difference in pitch. The male larynx accentuates its growth at puberty, increasing the length of the

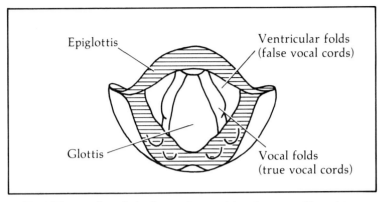

Fig. 5 The vocal cords in the resting position for normal breathing.

vocal cords which can be seen as the Adam's apple in the neck. As a result of these changes, the male voice becomes deeper.

The inability to speak (aphasia) is a distressing condition which may accompany a cerebral haemorrhage or cerebral thrombosis (CVA), or a cerebral tumour. Aphasia may be 'expressive'; that is to say, the patient is able to put his thoughts into words, but is unable to say them, no matter how hard he tries. In this type of aphasia, the lesion occurs in the left side of the brain of a right-handed person because the nerve fibres cross at the base of the brain. 'Receptive' aphasia is the failure to comprehend the spoken or written word; although words can be repeated, there is

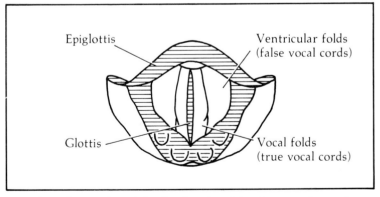

Fig. 6 The vocal cords in the closed position for normal speech.

no understanding of them. Communication for someone with hemiplegia and aphasia is further restricted by the paralysis, as he has lost the ability to substitute body language (signs and gestures) for speech.

Helping the aphasic patient

The elderly person with both expressive and receptive aphasia, following a stroke, poses an enormous challenge for nurses. When the patient first recovers consciousness, he will be confused and frightened by the strange surroundings and people. As recovery continues, he experiences anxiety, frustration and emotional lability, which leads to bouts of depression, anger, or sometimes inappropriate mirth. Initially, the nurse must anticipate his needs to reduce frustration. The patient with expressive aphasia, with adequate hearing, vision and intellect, is able to indicate his needs non-verbally, if offered a number of alternatives, e.g. a tray containing familiar items from which to choose; or asked short questions that can be answered with a nod, or shake of the head. Some typical questions are as follows:

1. Are you too hot/cold?
2. Would you like a drink?
3. Have you a headache?
4. Are you hungry?
5. Would you like your glasses?
6. Are you comfortable?
7. Do you want to go to the toilet?
8. Would you like to go to bed now?

The patient with receptive or mixed aphasia will not be able to co-operate because the problem is one of understanding, not expression. He needs to be given the opportunity to relate the article to its name, and requires constant repetition of the word whenever the same article is used. Some restoration of function usually occurs, but progress is often slow and impossible to predict, and is more difficult for elderly people with poor hearing or vision. The nurse will be mainly responsible for encouraging him to communicate his needs and fears, and it is important to discover the patient's previous level of ability, in speaking, hearing and seeing, from his family.

The following are some guidelines for the assessment of a patient with a loss of speech, in order to help rehabilitate him:

1. If a speech therapist is available to make a full assessment of the patient's ability, this is very useful in planning the

training programme, and encourages the patient that improvement is anticipated.

2. Where there is no speech therapist, the nurse must assess whether the patient can express his thoughts in writing or gestures.

3. The patient's level of understanding must be assessed. Does he understand what is said to him, in single words, or short sentences?

4. You must speak normally to the patient, regardless of the lack of response.

5. You must not assume that hearing and intelligence have also been lost, and do not discuss the patient as if he were not there.

6. You must address the patient by name, never use diminutives, or treat him as a child.

7. You must keep sentences short and relate them to the patient's current activity.

8. You should progress from single words to short sentences, and provide support and encouragement when frustration (or depression) occurs.

9. You should reinforce the spoken word by pictures, symbols or articles, in order to provide stimulation of the sensory pathways.

10. When giving physical care, such as a bath, articles in use should be named clearly. The patient should then be asked to repeat the word. Plenty of time must be allowed for a response.

11. You should keep the periods of instruction brief and free from tension.

12. You should involve relatives and friends in the retraining programme, so that, when the patient goes home, they can continue with the rehabilitation programme.

13. You should always approach the patient on the unaffected side when communicating with him.

SENSATION

Our skin contains receptors that are sensitive to pain, pressure, touch and temperature, relaying the information to the brain where it is interpreted. We are able to identify the shape, texture and composition of objects in our surroundings by touch, and to protect ourselves from harm by interpreting and acting upon the warning messages sent to the brain by the skin receptors.

In older people, the skin thins and loses its elasticity, becoming wrinkled and dry. Loss of sensation is not necessarily part of ageing, but some old people do have marked loss of sensation as a result of disorders of the nervous system that interfere with the transmission of the messages to the brain. As a result, they are unable to take the necessary precautions when handling hot dishes or pans, sitting too close to a fire, or stepping into a hot bath. For this reason no one with impaired sensation should ever be given a hot water bottle in bed, for serious burns may result.

We can help to overcome some of the dangers of sensory loss in older people by teaching them how to handle pots and pans safely, to use a bath thermometer to test the temperature of water, to protect the legs from direct heat when sitting in front of the fire, and to examine skin, particularly the feet, for signs of pressure, as well as stressing the importance of changing position at regular intervals.

TOUCH

By touching we are able to communicate our affection, empathy and understanding, and it is an important component of care when we are nursing someone with a sudden loss of speech, sight or hearing. If handling is firm and gentle, then comfort and reassurance are offered, which help to minimise the patient's fear and anxiety.

A patient who is expressing anger or frustration may be helped by someone who sits quietly, perhaps holding his hand, until the episode is over. Such action will indicate that his reaction is understood, even though it may not be considered the best way of overcoming the problem.

Dislike, disapproval, resentment and anger may also be expressed by the way we touch people when giving care; we must be aware of our feelings when we are helping someone to dress, walk, bathe or eat, and endeavour to remember that their disability prevents them walking away from us, and that they are sometimes totally dependent upon us for their physical, emotional and psychological well-being.

Some people like to be touched, others do not, so nurses must be alert for signs that touching is not acceptable to the patient and should respect his wishes. To do otherwise increases anxiety and tension.

NON-VERBAL COMMUNICATION

Body language is an important component of communication, and its value is not fully utilised as an indicator of mood and general health. We express our feelings and our relationship with others by the way we walk, sit or stand. A nurse who attempts to communicate with a patient when standing over him, demonstrates her authority as well as the patient's dependence, and does not encourage confidence or trust.

Facial expression can convey approachability and friendliness, or warn that such overtures are not welcome. Older people with poor sight cannot respond because they are unable to see features clearly or to make eye contact. Tone of voice is more important in conveying our mood to them. On the other hand, when meeting deaf people, expression, particularly eye contact, is very important in making our mood and meaning clear.

The Latin race are reputed to 'talk with their hands', and most of us do use gestures, hand movements or shrugs, to add emphasis to our words, or to contradict what we are saying. We may smile and say we do not mind when asked to perform a service for someone or to work late, but our posture and eyes may reveal that we are irritated, resentful or angry, and we may refuse to meet the other's eyes. We are unable to control non-verbal language in the same way as we censor speech. By studying our patients' non-verbal cues, we may be able to help them to overcome some of the problems they cannot or do not express to us.

SUMMARY

Ageing brings with it many disabilities but perhaps none is so limiting or cruel as the sensory loss which inhibits normal communication. Loneliness, isolation and despair threaten those who suffer severe sensory deprivation, and are a matter of great concern for those who seek to care for someone who is afflicted. Loss of hearing cuts one off from normal conversation, the radio and television, theatre and music. Loss of sight restricts freedom of movement, reading, handicrafts and hobbies, and speech loss prevents expression of thoughts, pleasure or needs. Loss of one sensory function can be ameliorated by developing another – for example, many blind people have very acute hearing – but this substitution and adaptability diminish with age, particularly when accompanied by lack of energy owing to frailty or illness.

For an aphasic person with poor hearing and failing vision, the environment is devoid of stimulation unless we are able to introduce additional material.

Grandchildren should be encouraged to hug their grandparents, because they do so naturally and spontaneously. Flowers and plants with strong perfumes and interesting textures may help elderly people to recall a much loved garden, and fresh fruit and vegetables will remind them of their gardening days. Boredom may be overcome by varying the day's routine – short walks can be arranged at differing times to gain the best of the weather, for example. Also the elderly person can sit in a different room each day.

Pets should be encouraged, for they communicate their affection and loyalty without words, and respond to kindness and warmth. It is believed that stroking animals can be therapeutic for elderly people. All our actions should be aimed at preserving the social contacts of the handicapped person, involving them in the daily living activity of the family, or institution, with kindness and humour.

8
NUTRITION AND DIET FOR THE ELDERLY

SUE THOMAS
Senior Dietitian,
St James's Hospital, Balham, London

Many of the myths surrounding the dietary needs of the elderly have been shattered in recent years. Amongst them was the mistaken belief that old people needed less food and that they should be provided with a 'geriatric diet' containing bland or even puréed food! But what are the dietary needs of the elderly? It is true that they need less energy (calories) than younger adults, but their requirement for all other nutrients changes little with ageing. Yet, for a variety of medical, social and environmental reasons, many old people have an inadequate diet, which causes sub-clinical malnutrition. There are few outward signs and symptoms of this condition and many old people can survive for months or even years in this state. However, if they meet with illness or injury, they may be too malnourished to meet the extra demands needed to make a swift recovery. This can lead to a rapid decline in health.

Table 7 lists the risk factors which may lead to poor nutrition in the elderly.

COMMON DIETARY PROBLEMS
Anaemia

Anaemia is the general term given to any condition where the oxygen-carrying capacity of the blood (haemoglobin) drops below normal. Whatever the cause of anaemia, the same symptoms are present in varying severity. These include tiredness, breathlessness, lack of energy and palpitations.

Iron-deficiency anaemia in old people is rarely caused by poor diet alone, but is usually found in association with chronic internal bleeding. It is treated with iron tablets or, in severe cases, by blood transfusion. Advice on increasing the iron content of the diet is always important. Good sources of iron include liver and liver products, such as pâté and liver sausage, kidney, red meats, corned beef, eggs, wholemeal bread, fortified breakfast cereals, lentils and green vegetables.

Anaemia caused by lack of folic acid, one of the B vitamins, is frequently caused by poor diet. Rarer causes of this type of anaemia are due to gastrointestinal disease and alcoholism. Rich sources of folic acid include liver and dark green leafy vegetables. As this vitamin is killed easily by prolonged cooking, elderly people who rely upon institutional catering, such as meals on wheels, or hospital diets, may have a deficient folic acid intake. Folic acid tablets and dietary advice are given to treat this anaemia.

Vitamin B12 deficiency, sometimes known as pernicious anaemia, is caused by the body's inability to produce a substance in the stomach, known as 'intrinsic factor', essential for the absorption of Vitamin B12 from the diet. This type of anaemia is more common with advancing age, and can be found also in people who have had gastric surgery in the past. In rare cases, Vitamin B12 deficiency has been found in people following vegan diets, which exclude all animal products. Pernicious anaemia is treated by monthly injections of Vitamin B12.

Vitamin C deficiency

Scurvy, caused by severe Vitamin C deficiency, is very rare nowadays, but has been reported occasionally amongst the elderly – in particular among old men living alone. However, a milder form of Vitamin C deficiency is common among the elderly, both in the community and in long-stay care. Signs and symptoms are difficult to detect, but may include an increased tendency to bruising, poor wound healing and, perhaps, listlessness.

Vitamin C deficiency is caused by lack of fresh vegetables and citrus fruits. It occurs in those housebound old people who are unable to get out to buy fresh food, and in those ignorant of their importance. As in the case of folic acid, people who rely on meals on wheels or institutional diets for their Vitamin C may also become deficient, because this vitamin is easily killed by lengthy cooking and by delays between cooking and consumption. In one recent meals-on-wheels survey, of people taking two meals on wheels per week, their Vitamin C intake was highest on the days

Table 7 Risk factors leading to poor nutrition in the elderly

1. Loneliness.
   a) Social isolation – living alone.
   b) Recent bereavement.
   c) Few or no outside interests.
2. Mental disturbance.
   a) Known psychiatric history.
   b) Confusional state.
   c) Senile dementia.
   d) Depression.
3. Physical disability.
   a) Being immobile or housebound.
   b) Arthritis, especially of hands.
   c) Being blind or partially sighted.
4. Effects of drugs.
   Causing nausea.
   a) Chemotherapy.
   b) Digoxin (heart tablets).
   c) Drugs for treatment of TB.
   Affecting vitamin and mineral status.
   a) Phenytoin and other anti-convulsants.
   b) Aspirin and anti-arthritic drugs (may cause anaemia through chronic blood loss).
   c) Water tablets (diuretics).
   d) Levodopa (treatment for Parkinson's disease).
5. Ignorance of nutrition.
   a) Widowers.
   b) Those eating only one meal per day.
   c) Pre-existing poor dietary habits.
   d) Obsessive ideas about food.
   e) Restricted variety of diet.
6. Impaired appetite.
   a) Following illness.
   b) Due to other factors, e.g. 1, 2, 4.
7. Economic position.
   a) Those existing on pension alone.
   b) Those with other high expenses e.g. heating, etc.
   c) Poor knowledge leading to poor choice and unwise use of available money.
8. Increased nutritional requirement.
   a) Those on bed rest.
   b) Those with bedsores.
   c) Pyrexia (especially long-term).
   d) Post-trauma, e.g. fall.
9. Poor dentition.
   No teeth, ill-fitting dentures or decayed teeth and bad gums.
10. Regular use of laxatives.
11. High alcohol intake.
    a) Leaving little money for food.
    b) Replacing meals.
    c) Causing impaired vitamin metabolism.
12. Recent discharge from hospital.

when they did not have meals on wheels! A quick way to assess whether there is enough Vitamin C in the diet is to find out whether the old person takes one of the following daily: fresh citrus fruit, e.g. orange or grapefruit, fresh fruit juice, freshly cooked greens or raw tomato. If he or she takes none of these, a deficiency should be suspected.

Useful sources of Vitamin C for the housebound, and for those not receiving regular supplies of fresh fruit and vegetables, include fortified blackcurrant juice, fortified instant fruit drinks and fortified instant mashed potato powder.

Vitamin D deficiency

From the age of 40 onwards there is a gradual loss of bone mineral from the body and thus, by the time old age is reached, bones may become quite brittle. This is a natural process of ageing for which there is little remedy, except to take regular exercise and adequate calcium in the diet (i.e. at least ½ pint of milk daily).

A more treatable bone condition caused by Vitamin D deficiency is seen occasionally amongst the elderly. This is known as osteomalacia, or adult rickets. Vitamin D transports dietary calcium from the gut to the bones, where it is used to strengthen them. Lack of Vitamin D prevents calcium from reaching the bones, and may lead to bone pain, muscle weakness and increased likelihood of falls and fractures. The chief source of Vitamin D in this country is derived from sunlight. Housebound old people, or those who dress from head to toe to brave the English summer, may be at risk of osteomalacia. We store Vitamin D during the sunny summer months and live on these stores throughout the winter months.

Osteomalacia can easily be prevented by adequate exposure to sunlight. Regular walks or rests in the sunshine, with rolled-up sleeves and open collars, will provide sufficient Vitamin D. Direct sunlight is not necessary – sitting in the shade will still be beneficial. It will be helpful for those who are housebound, or resistant to taking fresh air, to sit them on a balcony or near an open window. In homes and hospital, serving tea in the grounds is a good incentive to encourage residents to take advantage of sunshine!

Certain foods contain Vitamin D, and including these regularly in the diet will provide an extra boost of the vitamin, especially in the winter months when body stores are low. Good sources of

Vitamin D include: oily fish (e.g. herrings, kipper, mackerel, tuna fish), margarine, Ovaltine, liver, eggs and evaporated milk. Those old people who are housebound and unable to get into the sunshine, may benefit from Vitamin D tablets. However, it is unwise to buy these without medical advice because Vitamin D can be toxic if taken in large amounts.

Constipation

Constipation is a common complaint amongst the elderly. There is some confusion as to what the term actually means. 'Normal' bowel habits vary between different individuals – daily bowel motions may be normal for one person, whilst 2–3 bowel motions per week will be normal for another. Constipation occurs when the passage of waste matter is delayed in reaching the rectum, or when the rectum fails to empty completely. Pain and discomfort can follow. Constipation can cause loss of appetite and, in the already confused patient, agitation. In severe cases it can occasionally lead to bowel obstruction.

The four main factors causing constipation are lack of dietary fibre, lack of fluids, lack of exercise and the effects of medication. An adequate fibre intake to alleviate this should include the use of wholemeal bread, high fibre breakfast cereals and plenty of fresh fruit and vegetables. Wherever possible, leave the skin on potatoes, tomatoes and apples as this will also supply valuable fibre. Bran should be included in the diet if the high-fibre foods alone have not regulated bowel habits. Many old people believe that they need *less* fluids as they get older. They may even cut down on their fluid intake to reduce the urge to empty the bladder brought on by their use of water tablets (diuretics). An optimum fluid intake is 2–3 pints daily of water, tea, coffee or any other beverage. Simple advice for those people taking diuretics is to encourage them to drink more during the early part of the day and take their last drink at about 6 o'clock in the evening, thus ensuring that they will not be forced to get up in the night.

Old people should be encouraged to be as active as their physical capability will allow because exercise stimulates the tone of the bowel muscles. Attention to good diet, adequate fluids and exercise will all help to regulate bowel habits. The use of purgatives should be discouraged on a regular basis, as these can irritate the intestines, causing them to malabsorb some of the essential vitamins and minerals.

As has been mentioned earlier in this chapter, the dietary needs of the elderly differ little from those of younger adults. Their energy (calorie) requirement, however, is reduced, and this must be borne in mind when planning menus. Many old people, as they reduce their energy intake, also cut down on their intake of other, more essential nutrients. Menus should be planned to incorporate foods of a nutritionally high quality, and those containing little nutritive value, such as sugar and sugary foods, should be avoided. An excess of fried food with a high energy value should also be discouraged. For those with little appetite, small frequent meals are more suitable than the traditional three meals a day.

The belief that the elderly enjoy bland foods is wrong. With ageing, the senses of taste and smell may decline and the frequent complaint that 'food does not taste like it used to' may be a reflection of taste and smell impairment, rather than the fault of the diet of the 1980s! Experiment with stronger flavours and aromatic foods, such as curries and chilli con carne, and add them to the menus. The more liberal use of herbs and spices in cooking may also tempt the jaded palate. However, extra salt should not be used as it may counteract the good effects of any diuretics the patients may be taking.

Flexibility in menu planning is important, in order that seasonal luxuries, such as strawberries and cream, can be incorporated into the menu. If catering managers could allow for beer and sandwiches for male patients on Cup Final Day, or cream teas in the grounds on sunny Sunday afternoons, the patients' interest in food might be stimulated by such variety.

Lack of, or ill-fitting, dentures may cause an elderly person to self-select a soft diet, which is likely to be badly balanced. Referral to a dentist should be considered for all old people with inadequate dentition, although some are happier to do without teeth.

Menus should be planned carefully to take into consideration those old people with poor dentition, or other feeding problems. A soft, moist choice on the menu should be suitable for patients with feeding problems and is an appetising alternative to the purée diet, so often regarded as a 'geriatric food'! In rare cases, a medical condition, such as motor neurone disease, may prevent a person from swallowing even a soft diet; in these instances nourishing fluids should be offered (see Table 8).

Table 8 Supplements for those who need building up

1. *Fortified milk*. Add 2 level tablespoons milk powder to each pint of milk. Use this in all drinks, such as tea, coffee, cocoa, Ovaltine, on breakfast cereal and in cooking.
2. *Complan* made with milk, rather than water.
3. *Build-up* made with milk.
4. *Milkshake*. 1 pint cold milk, 1 level tablespoon milk powder and 2 small brickettes ice cream. Flavour with milkshake syrup, Camp coffee or liquidised tinned fruit.
5. *Egg nog*. ½ pint warm milk, 1 raw egg and 2 teaspoons sugar whisked together. Flavour with vanilla essence or a drop of brandy or sherry.
6. *Fruit juice*. Try either packet fruit juice or powdered fruit juice. Add a teaspoon of sugar or glucose to each glass.
7. *Milk jelly*. Make jelly with evaporated milk.
8. *Milk pudding*. Add 1 dessertspoon milk powder to tinned rice, or even tinned custard.
9. *High protein soup*. Either packet soup made with milk *or* tinned soup and 1 dessertspoon milk powder whisked in. 1 oz grated cheese can be sprinkled over each bowl before serving.
10. *In between meal snacks:* (a) Digestive biscuits and cheese. (b) Small sandwiches with a tasty filling such as ham, cold chicken, beef, corned beef, liver sausage, salami, tuna fish and lemon juice, cheese and pickle, cream cheese and cucumber, egg, banana or Marmite. (c) A small carton of plain or fruit yoghurt.

Sharing meals with others makes eating a social event. Communal dining, whether it be in a hospital, luncheon club or a family meal at home, may improve the ageing appetite. Attention to the dining environment is important. Tablecloths and flowers can add style to a dining area. Small portions of attractively served food will encourage the appetite, and the diner can always come back for a second helping if desired. The polite segregation of the messy eater may save embarrassment on all sides. Allow the slow eaters time to enjoy their meals without being rushed.

If a patient has to dine in bed make sure that he or she is sitting in an upright position, supported by plenty of pillows, with an adjustable trolley table conveniently placed for eating. Feeding of dependent patients is a time-consuming task, but if done with understanding, it will maintain the patient's good nutrition, and strengthen the bond between patient and nurse.

Special diets have a limited role amongst the elderly. Reducing diets should be considered only when obesity hinders the patient's recovery, or when staff find the patient too heavy to nurse efficiently. Such diets should exclude sugar, and food containing sugar, initially, as these contain 'empty' calories and few essential nutrients. If stricter advice is needed, a dietitian should be consulted so that the patient's diet can be carefully planned in order to provide high nutritive value, whilst restricting calories.

Elderly diabetics who are treated by diet only, or by diet and tablets, can be controlled adequately by being instructed to eat regularly, and to avoid all sugar and sugar-containing foods. However, for diabetics requiring insulin injections, a more detailed diet is needed. For those elderly patients who need building up after an operation or illness, or to aid the healing of bedsores, the use of extra nourishing fluids and snacks will help to boost the protein and energy intake (see Table 8).

In rare cases, tube-feeding may be considered necessary during acute illness, or following surgery, when the patient's appetite is poor and his nutritional status is critical. The decision to tube-feed should be made only after discussion with the whole medical team and, where possible, with the patient himself. Fine-bore naso-gastric tubes should be chosen and the feeding regime discussed with the dietitian.

Vitamin tablets are not necessary for healthy old people. However, if there are signs of vitamin deficiency, or if vitamin requirement is increased to help wound healing, a short vitamin course may be prescribed in hospital.

Further reading

Davies, L., *Easy Cooking for One or Two* (Penguin Handbooks, 1972), (also Magna Print Books).

Davies, L., *Three Score Years . . . and Then?* (Heinemann, 1981).

9

REHABILITATION AND MOBILITY

ROWENA KINSMAN

District Physiotherapist,
Barnet Health Authority, London

Rehabilitation of the elderly patient is an exciting challenge for all those concerned. It embraces the whole person, not just the clinical recovery of a particular part of the body. A young person may break his leg, which, when the plaster is removed, looks and feels 'shaky'. He will rehabilitate quickly and requires little effort from hospital staff. However, the elderly patient is different, for, if he breaks his leg, he may have other complicating pathologies, such as arthritis, chronic bronchitis, or a stroke. Whatever these are, the elderly person has learnt to accept and adapt to them. In the example used of breaking a leg, it is important to look at the elderly person as a whole. This will include other pathologies, deformities and the patient's expectations. The patient may have arthritis, which could make it difficult to use underarm crutches, necessitating the use of a walking frame, which provides a wider base and, therefore, less strain on the arms. The arthritis may not have been a problem previously, but now needs to be taken into consideration. Besides the patient's own problems, the elderly patient in hospital often spends large amounts of time in bed or in a chair beside the bed. When the plaster is removed, the patient may be stiff and may find it difficult to move. The expression 'gone off his feet' is often applied to such patients. Undoubtedly physical inactivity, chronic disease and disability contribute to the deterioration in their physical condition. It is, therefore, not surprising that they have problems when it comes to rehabilitation.

Rehabilitation, when applied to the elderly, is concerned with the well-being of the person as a whole, not just the clinical recovery. For successful rehabilitation it is essential to have a

Basic functional activities			
	Date of assessment:		
Patient's name:			
Bed 1. Rolling from side to side.			
2. Moving up and down bed.			
3. Getting in and out of bed.			
4. Sitting on side of bed.			
Chair 5. Standing up.			
6. Sitting down.			
Standing 7. Standing unsupported (2 minutes).			
Walking 8. Walking forwards.			
9. Walking backwards.			
10. Upstairs.			
11. Downstairs.			
12. Turning.			
13. Open/close door.			
14. Pick up things from floor.			
15. Down to floor.			
16. Up from floor.			
Toilet 17. On/off.			
18. Manage toileting.			
Score 3 = Independent 2 = Independent with aid			
1 = Assistance required 0 = Impossible			
X = Not tested			

Fig. 7 A physiotherapist's assessment form, used to record basic functional activities.

team approach. Each member of the team should be aware of all the issues which influence how the patient will manage at home – the domestic, social, psychological and economic issues. To cover all aspects of rehabilitation it is necessary to assess the patient and identify attainable goals. Rehabilitation can then be planned in a realistic manner, and subsequent success be evaluated. The physiotherapist is one member of the rehabilitation team, which generally comprises the geriatrician, nurses, social worker, occupational therapist, physiotherapist, volunteers and others. The role of the physiotherapist is to assess, give advice to the

Range of movements							
Date:	Shoulders		Hips		Knees		Trunk
	L	R	L	R	L	R	
Extension							
Flexion							
Abduction							
Adduction							
Rotation							
Score 2 = Normal movement 1 = Limited movement 0 = No movement Note: shaded areas indicate no movement in that direction.							

Fig. 8 A 'range of movement' assessment form.

Muscle power						
	Date of assessment:					
	L	R	L	R	L	R
Biceps						
Triceps						
Abdominals						
Glutei						
Hamstrings						
Quadriceps						
Score 2 = Normal power 1 = Reduced power 0 = No power						

Fig. 9 A muscle power assessment form.

patient, family and others caring for the patient, to provide specialised treatment whenever indicated, and to educate the patient and others in the best methods of handling. The assessment is important, as it provides an understanding of the conditions affecting the patient, whilst taking into account the physical, psychological and social circumstances, and forms the basis on which treatment is planned.

ASSESSMENT

Generally, it is easiest to use a form, for the purpose of assess-

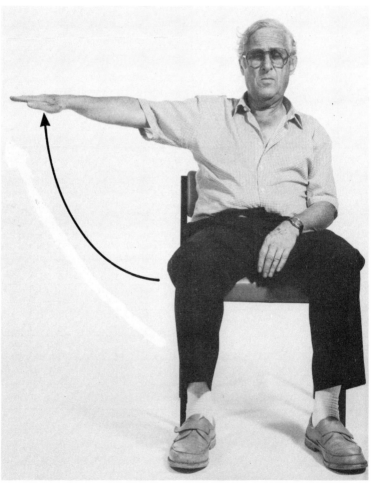

Photo. 1 Abduction – lifting a straight arm out to the side.

ment, that records basic functional activities, range of movement, and muscle power. The use of numerical scores enables the physiotherapist to make comparisons at subsequent assessments. Figure 7 allows the physiotherapist to make a functional

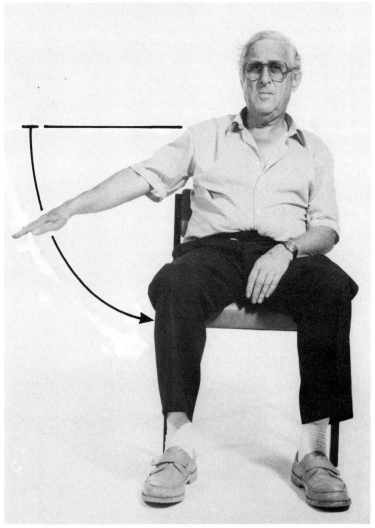

Photo. 2 Adduction – bringing a straight arm back to the side.

assessment of a patient. It is important that an assessment
gives an accurate picture as to how the patient performs and
whether an aid is used. The physiotherapist should assess
the patient's balance, too. That is, can the patient do the
following:

1. Sit unsupported. If not, how much support is needed?
2. Maintain balance, when pressure is applied to upset it.
3. Maintain balance, when attention is distracted.
4. Maintain standing balance.
5. Stand on either leg for a short period of time.

It is also necessary to check range of movement (see Fig. 8) and
muscle power (see Fig. 9). This is done by asking the patient to
perform movements, for example, abduction – to lift a straight
arm out to the side (see Photo. 1) and adduction – bring a straight
arm back to the side (see Photo. 2). If the patient has no difficulty,
or limitation with the movement, it is considered normal. Muscle
power is checked by applying a small amount of manual
resistance to the movement.

Throughout the assessment, the physiotherapist should
observe the quality of movement – does the patient move
smoothly, and are all movements integrated and co-ordinated? It

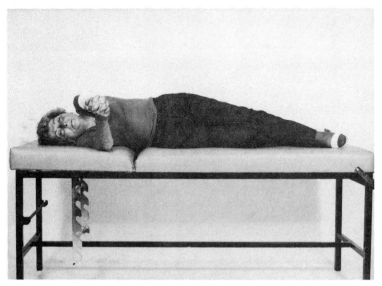

Photo. 3 A patient learns how to roll over in bed.

is important that the physiotherapist be aware of whether the patient is continent or not. Usually the management of incontinence is the concern of the nurses. Nevertheless a physiotherapist may have a special interest and, with her knowledge of muscle function and re-education, play a valuable part in the management of the incontinent patient. She can help train the patient to regain muscular control of the pelvic floor muscles. Whoever takes responsibility for the management of the incontinent patient should assess the patient carefully, in order that she has a very clear understanding of the pattern of incontinence. In consultation with the patient, a routine of toileting should be drawn up and acted upon. It is easier for the hospital staff if the patient is mobile and able to reach the toilet easily.

TREATMENT

Treatment is based on the assessment, and concentrates on those areas of poor performance. The physiotherapist may teach the patient how to roll over in bed (see Photo. 3). To do this it is necessary to know all the various components of movements involved, and then to identify where the patient has difficulty. Having identified this, it is necessary to teach the patient, through simple instructions, how to roll over, and to give opportunity for practice. This would involve teaching other members of the team how the patient can perform the activity. The therapist may break down an activity into simple stages – for example, rolling over – as follows:

1. I take my hands to my left.
2. I cross my right leg over my left.
3. I roll to my left.

Sometimes it is necessary to help the patient. When one helps a patient it is important to know why one is helping. In the example of 'rolling over to the left' the patient may, as a result of a stroke, have difficulty crossing one leg over the other, and will need help. This help should be just sufficient to enable the patient to achieve the desired movement. If there is too much help, the patient will come to rely on it and will not perform actively. Active movement is essential if the patient is going to learn how to function again. In this instance, the physiotherapist will help the patient to find the easiest way of rolling over, and will then show the other members of the multidisciplinary team, and the family, how the patient performs and how they can best help.

The patient learns each part, discarding some parts as they become known. In this way the patient is encouraged, and is often prepared to work for long periods of time. The therapist should take care to start with easy movements, gradually progressing to more difficult ones. Minimal assistance may be given whenever necessary. Gradually this is withdrawn until the patient is able to perform independently. This success in itself is motivating and, if rehabilitation is to succeed, it is essential to have the patient's co-operation and motivation.

The physiotherapist should pay particular attention to the patient's mobility and, if necessary, give exercises for the following reasons:

1. To increase the range of movement.
2. To mobilise and strengthen the back and trunk muscles.
3. To improve stability, so that the patient is better able to lift and lower his body weight.
4. To move easily from standing and sitting, and to maintain co-ordination during a change of positions.

Physiotherapists are often unable to spend much time with their patients, so it is important that they liaise with the other members of the multidisciplinary team, showing them what the patient can do, and what exercises he should practise. There are some units that are unfortunate in that they do not have any physiotherapy, and the nurses are left to cope as best they can. In these circumstances, the best advice is to study yourself and how you move. For instance, the patient who has difficulty getting in and out of a chair may have one or more of the following problems:

1. He cannot come forward on the chair with his buttocks.
2. He cannot put weight down through both feet.
3. He cannot lean forward.
4. He cannot push down on his hands.

It is necessary to decide which of the above are causing the problem and then to examine carefully how you yourself get out of a chair. This is done by performing the movement several times. Having ascertained the problem and the probable solution, you are in a position to help the patient.

The patient who has had a stroke may experience difficulty keeping both feet on the floor. This is because of associated movements that occur as a result of the stroke. There are two ways of dealing with this. One is to wedge the affected foot with one's own (see Photo. 4). The second is to teach the patient to take

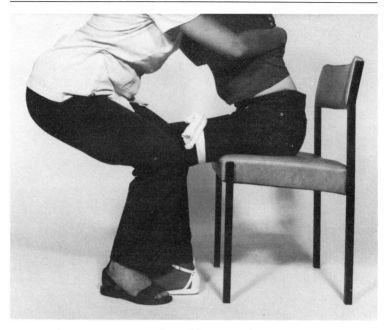

Photo. 4 A patient's affected foot is wedged between the physiotherapist's feet in order to help her to keep both feet on the ground.

the maximum weight down through the leg, in order that it cannot move.

When working with the elderly patient, the physiotherapist should be aware of the patient's general condition and tolerance to exercise. Patients can be divided into various groups as follows:

1. Slow-stream rehabilitation

These patients may be severely disabled and may be able to cope with only a little treatment at a time. For instance, the arthritic patient who suffers from a stroke is already handicapped by the arthritis and by much discomfort. As a result of the stroke, he must move in a different way, in order to give the affected side an equal chance of recovery. This patient benefits from short spells of treatment interspersed throughout the day.

2. Medium-stream rehabilitation

These patients may be independent, but are unsteady on their feet and have lost their confidence. Each one needs much treatment to strengthen the muscles. This rehabilitation could be part of a day programme and include both group work and individual treatment, with the emphasis being placed on helping the patient regain stability and confidence. This sort of treatment generally takes place in a day hospital, which the patient may visit daily initially, reducing his attendances as he improves.

3. Intensive rehabilitation

This is given to those patients who have a specific problem, for example a fracture. The patient may need a programme of intensive mobilisation in order to regain full function. This treatment may take place in a physiotherapy department. The physiotherapist assesses the patient and, in the light of this, decides upon a suitable course of treatment. So far the treatment described has been given in hospital; however, it is becoming increasingly more popular to treat the elderly patient in his home environment. This is, of course, more realistic, as the patient is used to his surroundings and can readily gauge appropriate distances, i.e. from one room to another. Generally, referral to community physiotherapy is through the general practitioner. The district nursing sister or health visitor may suggest to the general practitioner that the physiotherapist be asked to advise and, in some instances, to treat. Generally, community physiotherapy is of an advisory nature; that is, the 'carers' are shown how to handle the patient, how to help the patient achieve maximum function, and what the patient should practise or do for himself. In other words, the community physiotherapist is teaching the patient, and those caring for the patient, how to achieve optimal potential. The patient may then be visited at home to be given treatment, or advised on the best method of management. For example, when using a walking frame should the patient leave the frame at the bottom of the stairs and have another at the top of the stairs?

The community physiotherapist plays a valuable role by supporting patients in their own homes, often avoiding or delaying admission to hospital. It should be noted that there are district variations, with some community physiotherapists offering to undertake treatments, as well as acting in an advisory capacity.

The decision as to the type of service rests with the district physiotherapist, where there is one, and the health district management team. Each service will vary depending upon the character of the district, the availability of transport facilities and staff. Where there is a district physiotherapist, there is an opportunity to rationalise the service and make the most use of the available resources. Hospitals also use the community physiotherapy services – in particular to facilitate a patient's discharge.

ADVICE

The physiotherapist must advise all staff and family how the elderly patient performs the activities of daily living, and what functional level the patient has attained. For example, if the patient uses a walking aid, such as a walking frame, everyone involved should be shown how the patient should use it. The patient should take equal weight down through the arms. The frame is lifted and placed in front of the patient so that he can step towards the frame. All the feet of the frame should be flat on the floor. A problem often occurs when a patient tries to open a door (see Photo. 5) or to go through a doorway with a walking frame. The physiotherapist must ensure that the patient has sufficient balance to maintain his position whilst doing this. There is often a need to train the patient carefully to sit down on, and get out of, a chair (see Photo. 6). Going up and down a step (Photos 7 and 8) often presents problems, which are compounded if there are no banister rails, or only one. As a rule of thumb, the patient descends by placing the weak leg down first and then bringing the stronger leg to it. When going upstairs, it is the stronger leg that leads. The choice of leg is really common sense, for the leg that has to do most of the supporting must be in a position to do so. There are some instances where stepping down one step at a time is impossible, or the patient needs to step sideways, or even backwards. The physiotherapist advises on the best method and demonstrates this to all relevant carers.

Often it is necessary to advise about footwear. All too often elderly patients wear slippers that are floppy, giving no support. The elderly foot becomes sensitive to ill-fitting footwear – probably why old people resort to slippers. Most districts have a district chiropodist service. Unlike physiotherapy, chiropodists work predominantly in the community. Unfortunately, these services are hard-pressed, nevertheless problems should be

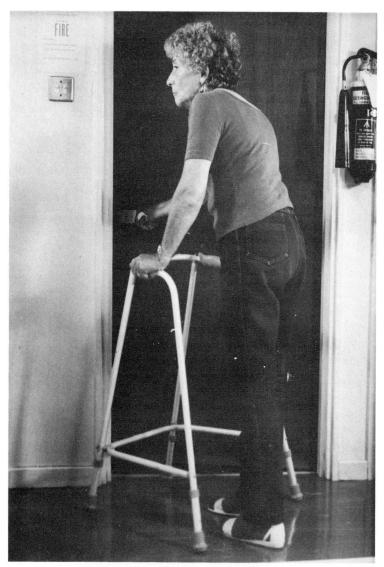

Photo. 5 A patient learns how to open a door when using
a walking frame.

referred to this service. Many manufacturers are aware of the problems, and a variety of shoes are now available so that elderly patients need be uncomfortable no longer. The Disabled Living Foundation will give advice on manufacturers, styles of shoes, and effective care. Physiotherapists can be involved in advising the family about the most suitable layout of the furniture at home. Often elderly patients live in overcrowded rooms, and it is necessary, being tactful, to point out that they would manage more independently without, for instance, loose carpets or clutter. Sometimes it may be best for the patient to change his bed or the bed height.

Physiotherapists can be involved in the provision of aids, most commonly walking aids. There are a variety of walking aids on the market, and many different organisations are prepared to

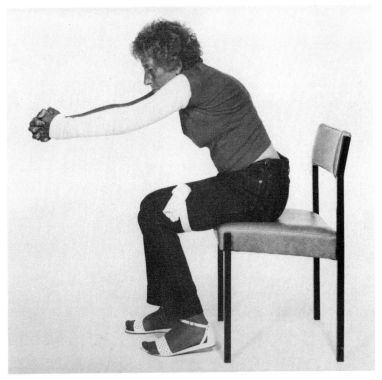

Photo. 6 A patient is trained to sit down on, and get out of, a chair.

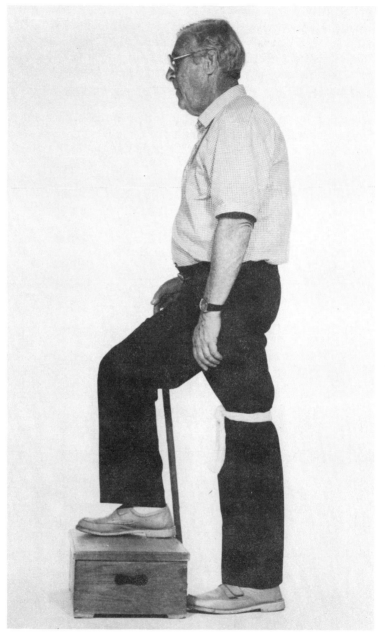

Photo. 7 A patient learns how to go up a step. (The stronger leg leads.)

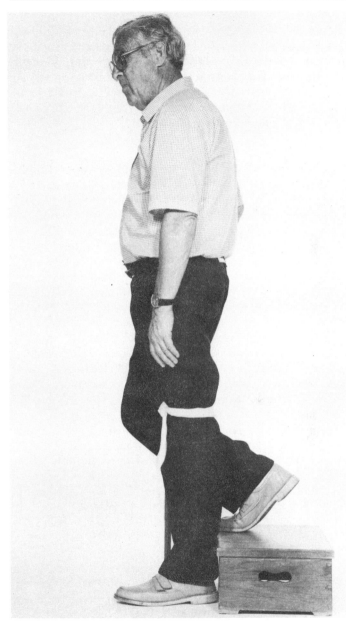

Photo. 8 A patient learns how to come down a step.
(The weaker leg leads.)

make one-off adaptations to these aids. Again, the DLF can be approached for such advice. The aids should be simple and suit the patient's needs. It must be borne in mind, when considering an aid, that you are giving the patient a 'prop' and, wherever possible, this should be considered as a temporary measure. The therapist should show the support staff how to maintain the equipment, for example pumping up the tyres of the wheelchair, and how a piece of equipment is to be used.

HANDLING

The physiotherapist must be certain that those supporting the elderly person know how to handle him. In hospital this is important, for it is often possible to facilitate the patient's recovery through careful handling. If one pauses for a moment to think how one moves forward in a chair, one realises that the weight is taken on one buttock whilst moving the other forward, until one is at the edge of the chair. Often the patient needs only minimal help to relearn this activity. The physiotherapist teaches all those handling the patient, in order that the patient can achieve maximal function. Besides this, it is important that supporting staff and family be aware of the best way of handling, so as to prevent complications; for example, the stroke patient is liable to develop a painful shoulder. This can be prevented by teaching the patient how to assist the affected arm, and by teaching others how to hold the shoulder. That is done by placing a hand in the armpit, lifting the whole of the affected shoulder and ensuring that there is no downward pull (see Photo. 9). It is the downward pull, which puts a stretch on weak shoulder muscles, that can bring about a painful shoulder.

It would be incomplete, when discussing handling, not to discuss how those supporting the elderly patient should prevent harming their own backs. This is important, as back pain is often the cause of breakdown in the support system of the elderly patient. With care, there is no need to strain the back. The supporters should be taught to keep their backs in the correct position, bending at the hips and knees, with their backs straight. It is a useful tip to lift one's head before starting to lift, as this automatically gets the back into the correct position. The support-ers should be shown where to place their feet – on either side of the patient's feet or in front of the affected foot – so that the patient's feet are wedged and cannot slip.

All those working with the elderly should be taught to care for

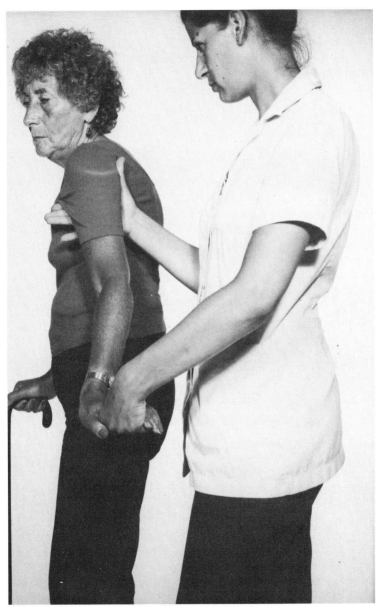

Photo. 9 A physiotherapist helping on the affected side of
a hemiplegic patient.

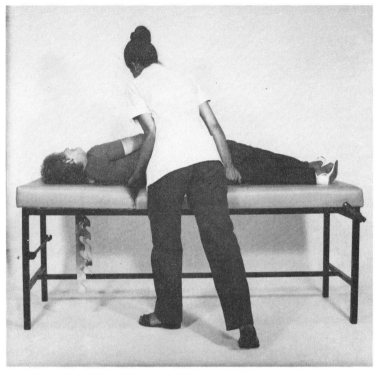

Photo. 10 A carer should have a straight back when assisting an elderly person to roll over in bed.

their backs at all times. It is easiest to do this if one has a clear understanding of correct posture. Good posture involves carrying the body weight evenly over the heels and the outer borders of the feet, with the toes slightly gripping the floor. The knees are slightly bent and the pelvis should be tilted so that the buttocks are tucked under and the stomach flat. The shoulders should be back and slightly raised, with the head balanced on the shoulders in mid-position and the chin tucked in. This posture should be maintained for all activities. It thus becomes obvious that, in order to maintain the posture of the back when lifting, it is necessary to bend at the hips and knees. Similar consideration should be given to posture when helping a patient to roll over in bed, to get out of a chair, or to get in and out of a bath. Carers should never lift without thinking of why they are lifting, where they are lifting to, and how they can best achieve this. They should take into account distances to be moved, the weight of the object, and whether or not it can be held close to the body (see Photos 10, 11 and 12).

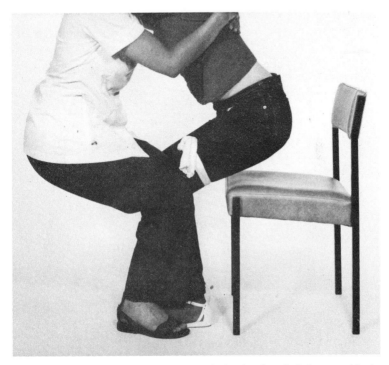

Photo. 11 A carer should have a straight back when helping an elderly person to stand up.

CONCLUSION

The physiotherapist, as a member of the multidisciplinary team, should regularly assess the patient, reporting problems back to the team, and co-ordinating treatment with other team members. At the time when the decision to withdraw the rehabilitation services is made, it is important to have a discharge summary of the patient's level of performance. A follow-up assessment, in order to ensure that the patient has maintained his progress, is

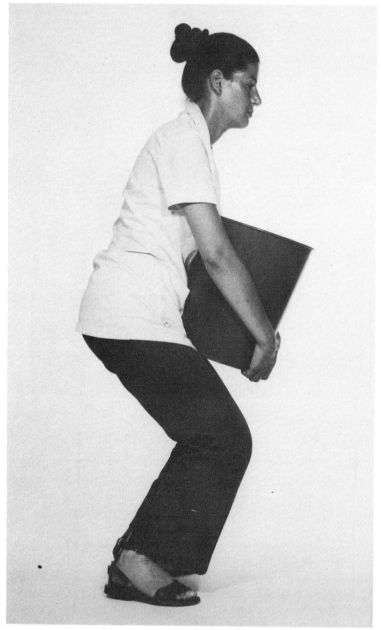

Photo. 12 A carer should lift heavy weights with a straight back.

also necessary. Sometimes, however, it is not possible to discharge a severely disabled person, as he may need regular
maintenance within a totally supportive environment, i.e. a long-
term ward. At whatever level of care deemed appropriate by the
team, the physiotherapist will be closely involved.

10
OCCUPATIONAL THERAPY FOR THE ELDERLY

ANNE DUMMETT
District Occupational Therapist,
Islington Health Authority, London

The occupational therapist has a contribution to make in the field of geriatrics which is far greater, and goes considerably further, than helping individuals pass the time. An illuminating definition of occupational therapy is: 'assessment and treatment of temporarily or permanently disabled people (physically or psychiatrically diseased) through the specific use of selected activity'. The purpose is to prevent disability, to improve health and to fulfil the person's needs by achieving optimum function and independence in his work, social and domestic environment. To achieve these objectives, an occupational therapist undertakes a three-year training that covers medicine and psychiatry. He or she acquires a practical competence in a wide range of activities (such as pottery, printing, social skills, activities of daily living), and undertakes a year's clinical practice in hospitals and the community, acquiring knowledge and expertise over as full a range of medical and psychiatric conditions as possible.

The occupational therapist has the opportunity of using the widest variety of his or her skills with the elderly. The pace may be slower than working with other groups, but there is time for assessment and problem-solving in a truly multidisciplinary environment. For those who have a sudden disability, for example after a stroke, new techniques have to be learned so that familiar tasks can be achieved. Families will have to cope with the changed circumstances, too, and the fear of possible recurrences of illness. If a wife becomes severely disabled and the husband does not know how to cook, he will have to learn this skill.

Similarly, if a husband becomes ill, the wife may have to learn about the financial aspects of their life, or how to deal with tax returns, if she has not had to cope with these before.

Elderly people who have been bereaved can become acutely depressed, which can place them at risk. The occupational therapist spends a large part of her work with the elderly and, by early intervention, can help maintain independence and provide support to relatives or carers at times of crisis. The support provided is invariably in conjunction with hospital personnel, social workers, home helps, district nursing sisters and other colleagues. This is to ensure that, wherever resources are available, the elderly person can take the best advantage of them.

It is important to ensure that any work the therapist has done to facilitate independence is enhanced and encouraged by everyone. The occupational therapist has a teaching role and a role of communication *vis-à-vis* nursing staff, medical staff, other therapists, relatives and, most importantly, the individual himself. Her prime task is to find out what an individual is able to do, in spite of his disability. She must ascertain whether the elderly person (e.g. who has suffered a stroke, is continually overbalancing or is depressed through bereavement) can dress himself, manage to wash and go to the toilet, make a hot drink, get in and out of bed (see Photo. 13) or get up and down from a chair. These are activities that an able-bodied person takes for granted, but a disabled person finds impossible to cope with. The occupational therapist will see how an individual manages and then advises and teaches easier methods, or supplies simple aids to assist. In addition to these tasks, or 'activities of daily living', an occupational therapist will create activities to stimulate social interactions and mental functions, and to refresh people's interests.

The occupational therapist in the multidisciplinary team is able to indicate how well, and at what level of independence, an older person can manage – whether he can return home, will require help from the social services, in the form of meals on wheels, because he cannot manage the more complex tasks of shopping and cooking, or requires constant support. She discovers this by carrying out a home-visit, either prior to the patient returning home from hospital or when he is at home. It is important that she does the following:

1. She reassures the patient that he will be able to cope at home or suggests ways in which a patient can cope.

2. She determines whether a mildly confused patient becomes more rational at home, amongst familiar surroundings.
3. She discusses the provision of aids and adaptations or methods of working suitable for the patient in his environment.
4. She involves caring relatives and others in order that their worries can be discussed, and dealt with, or alleviated.

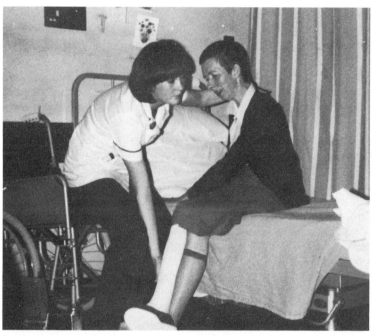

Photo. 13 An occupational therapist teaches a patient a method of getting on and off her bed.

The types of elderly patients most frequently seen by an occupational therapist are stroke patients, amputees, arthritics, orthopaedic and surgical cases (in particular people with broken femurs, hip replacements or broken wrists), patients with heart and chest problems, or balance problems, the elderly mentally ill (a varied range of mental illness, both acute and chronic, are included here, i.e. depression after bereavement or chronic schizophrenia), and psychogeriatrics.

THE ELDERLY IN HOSPITAL

With the increasing number of elderly people in the population a greater proportion of them require hospital treatment. The essential role of the occupational therapist is to retain the elderly person's independence as long as possible. Patients may be referred from their own homes, residential or sheltered accommodation, or from within the hospital. The occupational therapist is sometimes requested to do a home assessment, in order to *prevent* hospital admission. Her aim is to assess how the individual is managing within his own environment, and whether treatment or provision of aids could prevent unnecessary admission. In many cases another colleague, i.e. nurse, social worker or physiotherapist, may accompany the occupational therapist.

A typical case is an elderly person who has been continually falling, either out of bed, or around his home. The problems may have arisen because the person has stress incontinence – he cannot reach the toilet in time and, in his anxiety not to wet himself, rushes and trips over a rug or tumbles from a high bed. The provision of a commode in the bedroom, the removal of loose rugs, the re-arrangement of furniture to act as 'staging posts', as well as counselling the patient, may ease the situation considerably. A nurse or physiotherapist can treat this stress incontinence at the patient's home, so that he does not have to go into hospital.

The aim of the occupational therapist working in a hospital is to assess and treat, enabling the maximum level of independence to be achieved. This avoids dependency, and maintains quality of life for the individual within the community, hospital or residential unit. As a member of the treatment team, her specialist knowledge of domestic skills, activities of daily living, and cerebral function, contribute towards the treatment of the patient.

In order to help establish the level of cerebral function, a test can be carried out (see Fig. 10). This helps the team plan treatment and, in part, defines how confused a patient is. An elderly man who may be labelled 'senile dement' or 'very confused' by members of staff will be given this test repeatedly, over a period of time. In many cases the 'confusion' is due to the fact that he is in a different environment. Once the patient has adapted and settled, he becomes less 'confused', and functions at his usual level.

Simple tests of cerebral function	

Name .... Age .... Ward........

Date of admission .... Right- or left-handed.............

Date test performed .... Time ....

Observer's name..

Tests	Score

Memory
1. Name. 2 1 0
2. Age. 2 1 0
3. Address or last address before admission.
   (Q. Where did you live before you came into hospital?) 2 1 0
4. Ask patient to remember address – enquire after 10 minutes exactly. 5 4 3 2 1 0

Vocabulary
5. Define the meaning of: ship, fabric, remorse, reluctant, sanctuary. 5 4 3 2 1 0

Calculation
6. Subtract 17½p from 50p. 2 – 0

Orientation
7. State time of day (morning, afternoon or evening). 1 0
8. State whereabouts (room or hospital). 1 0

Speech
9. Name objects on a tray. Five should be held up separately – coin, button, pencil, key and scissors. 5 4 3 2 1 0
10. Obey simple commands e.g. 'Put out your tongue'. 1 0
11. Read simple instructions e.g. 'Raise your arms'. Can instructions be obeyed? 1 0
12. Read aloud. 1 0
13. Write name spontaneously. 1 0

Practical tests
14. Copy patterns with right hand using three matchsticks. 1 0
15. Copy patterns with left hand using three matchsticks. 1 0
16. Copy patterns with right hand using five matchsticks. 1 0
17. Copy patterns with left hand using five matchsticks. 1 0

Toy tests
18. Posting box. 6 5 4 3 2 1 0
19. Pyramid rings. 6 – 4 – 2 – 0

Check answer to memory test (question 4).

Total score [ ]

To score: circle the appropriate figure under the 'score' column, according to the patient's ability to get the answer, or parts of the answer, right. Add up the score at the end.

The therapist may be involved in ensuring that the ward environment fosters independence. For example, she may advise the hospital on appropriate chairs, wheelchairs, special equipment in toilets or bathrooms, or appropriate heights of furniture or rails, for the wards. Some examples of helpful equipment are: a Manoy chair in differing heights with lumbar supports, a Parker Knoll geriatric chair, different types of bath rails, a bathboard or bathseat, and a raised toilet seat. Aids for individual patients may be supplied by hospital therapists, but they are given more commonly to the individual going home, or to a home, by social services community occupational therapists. Where adaptations to the home are necessary – a stair lift for a severe rheumatoid arthritic to get to the upstairs bathroom and bedroom, or a ramp for a wheelchair-bound individual – the social services community occupational therapist will be involved.

If the family understand the elderly relative's capabilities, and have been instructed by the therapist in the ways they can provide help, then maximum co-operation is likely to be achieved. An awareness of how they can best help themselves should be included in this education, i.e. avoiding back strain by having bathing aids, or having the names of agencies to call in a crisis.

The occupational therapist carries out an assessment to ascertain the nature and extent of the problems (see Fig. 11). A treatment programme is established, according to the needs of the individual and will be modified, reviewed and re-assessed frequently. The treatment will concentrate on personal, physical, psychological, social and domestic needs, the aim being to restore the individual to his or her maximum ability. The complexity of social, psychological and physical factors contributes in some, perhaps all, of the following areas: personal independence, domestic skills, physical problems, and social and leisure activities. Whatever the prognosis may be, personal independence is a priority.

On admission to hospital, well-established patterns of behaviour are disturbed. This can affect bodily functions, sometimes contributing to incontinence or constipation. Disturbance of sleeping and eating patterns may increase confusion, and may lead to frustration. The treatment team will work together to achieve a basic level of independence, so that patients can perform essential daily tasks – for example, moving about the

Fig. 10 A cerebral function assessment form.

bed, from bed to chair, walking or wheeling themselves to the bathroom and toilet, dressing and feeding themselves. An occupational therapist knows that patients achieve these tasks at different paces, and that it is important to allow enough time for them to master difficulties. For example, it is important to allow an elderly person to dress himself, and practise this (providing aids, if necessary), than have everything done for him.

In many instances the therapist will advise other staff on methods by which the task is more easily achieved. She may devise a specific programme with other therapists – physiothera-

Functional assessment		
Name .... Rating scale	1 = Totally independent.	3 = Needs assistance.
Record no. .... Date	2 = Independent with aids.	4 = Totally dependent.

1. Mobility
Walking – on own
       – with aid
Wheelchair
Stairs
Car
Public transport
Transfers
Bed   – on
        – off
Chair   – on
        – off
Bath   – in
        – out
Toilet – on
        – off
 	
2. Clothing
Undressing – lower
            – upper
Dressing   – lower
            – upper
Fastenings
Zip
Buttons
Velcro
Socks/stockings
Shoes
Splint
 	
3. Self care
Washing
Bathing
Toilet
Make-up
Shaving
Hair
 	
4. Eating and drinking
Knife and fork
Fork
Spoon
Cutting food
Cup/glass
	5. Cooking
	Lifting saucepan
	Filling kettle
	Vegetable preparation
	Opening jars
	Opening tins
	Make and pour tea
	Meal – 1 course
	        – 2 courses
	Washing up
	Drying up
	Shopping
	
	6. Household
	Housework – light
	             – heavy
	Laundry
	Ironing
	
	7. Safety
	Cooker – gas
	        – electric
	Hob – light
	       – use
	Grill – light
	       – use
	Heating – turn on
	         – turn off
	
	8. Communication
	Dysphasia
	Aphasia
	Able to read
	Able to write
	Use telephone
	Handle money
	
	9. Mental and physical
	    state
	Orientation
	Memory
	Attitude
	Mood
	Hearing
		Vision
		Balance
		Co-ordination
		(rate as
		good-poor, 1–4)
		
		10. General activities
		Use of keys
		Lights
		Pick up self
		  from floor
		Pick up objects
		Bolt and
		  unbolt door
		Open and
		  close windows
		Strike match
		Manage a meter
		Open and close
		  cupboards
		
		11. Children
		Feed
		Wash
		Dress
		Pushchair
		Transport
		
		12. Home situation
		(tick as appropriate)
		House – private
		          – council
		Flat – private
		          – council
		Part III home
		Lives – alone
		         – with family
		         – with friends
		         – others

Fig. 11 An occupational therapist's functional assessment form.

pists or speech therapists – to overcome particular problems, i.e. of mobility or of verbal communication. For instance, when a stroke patient is absorbed in a creative activity, such as cooking, he may use familiar expressive speech which would not be used during a formal speech therapy session.

An elderly person living at home, perhaps alone, or alone for the greater part of the day, must be able to go shopping, prepare and cook a meal, make a hot drink and carry out necessary household tasks. Initially the occupational therapist may ask the patient to prepare a hot drink (either for herself or a group). Then, as familiar tasks are achieved, the patient can progress to other tasks within his or her capability. Preparing vegetables, laying the table, or washing dishes, can contribute to a 'home routine' programme.

Other activities, such as walking over rough ground (see Photo. 14), using public transport, knowing the highway code, and shopping may also be included in such a programme. In some cases, independence in some household skills cannot be achieved, and a home help, or meals on wheels, will have to be provided. In addition, other social services, such as attendance at a luncheon club or day centre, may be arranged to prevent isolation or loneliness.

The elderly patient will be taught to use such aids as built-up handles on cutlery or knives, and adapted cutting boards or jar openers (see Photo. 15). If these are not provided, a new way of performing a task will be taught.

Each elderly person makes social contact in a different way. He may want to be able to listen and talk to others, feel useful, or just be left alone. Through the earlier devised daily programme, the occupational therapist creates a situation in which patients are encouraged to gain confidence and self-esteem. Aids can be provided to help with leisure pursuits, hobbies and interests. Attendance at a day centre may be organised, or contact established with agencies such as adult educational institutes, in order to maintain social contacts when the patient is back at home.

THE ELDERLY MENTALLY ILL

Much of what has gone before is applied to psychiatrically ill patients, and treatment is directed towards routine, thus helping to avoid unnecessary confusion. Team work is essential in daily activities if the elderly person is to relate to them and benefit from

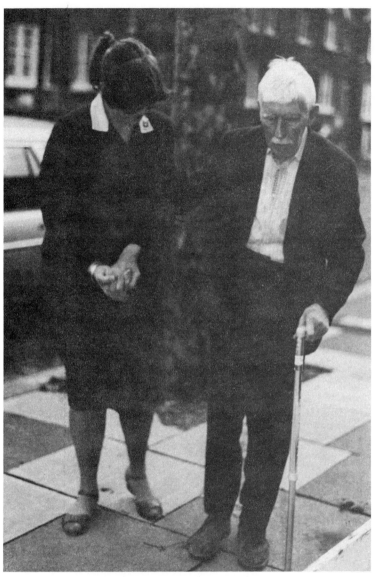

Photo. 14 An elderly person is helped to walk over rough ground.

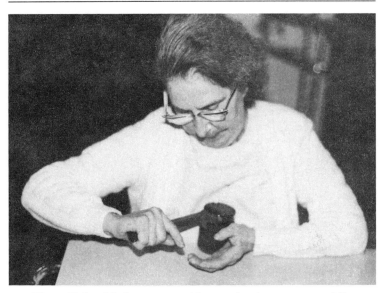

Photo. 15 An elderly person, with a weak grip, uses a specially
adapted jar opener.

the routine. To achieve this, considerable blurring of professional
roles occurs. A wide variety of treatment skills can be used with
the mentally ill, i.e. discussion groups, reality orientation and
supportive group psychotherapy. These activities help the
individual concentrate on specific subjects, thus establishing
concentration.

The objectives of an occupational therapy programme with the
elderly mentally ill are to be an aid to diagnosis and management
of the patient's mental function (particularly mood and
behaviour), to stimulate interest and motivate the patient, to
alleviate anxiety, agitation and confusion, to develop awareness
of self and others and promote social interaction, and to prevent
both mental and physical deterioration. Problems which may
occur in psychiatry include the recurrence of the illness in the
elderly, for example paranoia and depression. Often short-term
admission to hospital is required in these cases. Adjustment to
the deteriorating process of dementia poses considerable problems. Involvement in support groups for relatives, in addition to
a devised programme for the patient, then forms a part of the
occupational therapy programme.

THE ELDERLY IN CONTINUING CARE

Some elderly people are referred to continuing care wards as they are unable to become sufficiently independent, in spite of assessment and treatment. The occupational therapist will be involved in activity programmes which provide intellectual stimulation and physical activity. Creative projects will be devised to enable those with varying handicaps to make a valid contribution (see Photo. 16). There is endless scope for using creative or educative media, and for taking part in social activities, gardening and outings. Other members of the team, volunteers and relatives or outside agencies (i.e. art teachers, handicraft teachers) will also be involved, in order to give maximum participation.

THE ELDERLY IN THE COMMUNITY

Of the increasing number of elderly people, many do not go into hospital. They remain either in their own home, or go to live in a

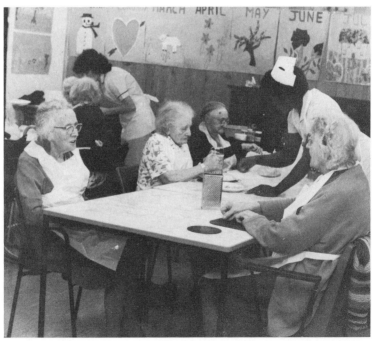

Photo. 16 Some elderly people preparing food as part of a creative project.

local authority home, or a private 'rest' home. As people get older they experience increasing difficulties with everyday activities, such as dressing or going to the toilet. In some cases such tasks become quite a struggle, or even hazardous. Due to ageing, the person may experience frequent loss of balance, made worse by incorrect heights of chairs, toilet or bed, and by little or nothing to hold on to to stabilise him.

The community occupational therapist will provide many of the following small appropriate aids which will enable the elderly individual retain his or her independence, and will reduce risk:

1. A commode, correctly positioned, and adjacent to the bed, to prevent a journey at night to a downstairs or outside toilet.
2. A bed downstairs to eliminate the danger of a bad fall on stairs.
3. A chair which is firm and comfortable for sitting in for lengthy periods. It should be of the correct height to prevent struggle (and thus possible fall or accident when getting up or sitting down).
4. Communication devices to the front door so that keys need not be left in the latch. These enable the elderly person to ascertain who is at the door before opening it and thus prevent unsolicited visitors, so that he or she feels more secure if living alone (see Photo. 17).
5. Dressing aids, i.e. elastic shoe laces, long-handled comb/shaver. Advice will also be given on appropriate clothing fastenings.
6. Bathing aids and rails to prevent falls and to alleviate relatives' anxiety, or prevent back injury to a carer who may be assisting.
7. Feeding aids, such as expanded handles on cutlery.

These aids and adaptations help the elderly to retain their self-confidence, dignity and independence.

There are resources within the community, such as day centres or homes providing day care, which offer a hot meal, company, a change of scene and sometimes a bath, and, perhaps of greatest importance, the opportunity for staff to keep in regular touch with those potentially at risk.

Unfortunately, a stage may be reached where an elderly person is unable to look after himself at home and a residential place is the only reasonable alternative. If the individual is well known to the occupational therapist, and contact with her in the home is retained, this will help the elderly person to adjust to the difficult transposition. Wherever possible, advice as to the necessary aids, and appropriate heights of beds, chairs, etc., will be given to the residential establishment, as well as the necessary information about his ability and level of independence. All this will help the elderly person to adapt to, and adopt, the new home more readily.

Some community occupational therapists work with the staff in homes in developing programmes aimed at increasing and maintaining independence of the residents, or providing mentally and physically stimulating activities. In some instances, an elderly person may stay in a 'home' for a protracted period, in order to increase his level of independence and thus restore his ability to return to his own home.

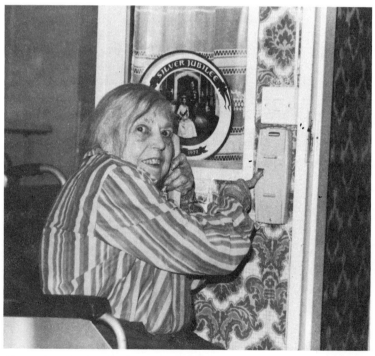

Photo. 17 An automatic door opening system. This is useful as it enables elderly people to identify their visitors before granting entry and, when confined to wheelchairs, to unlock their front doors by remote control.

Community occupational therapists may also be involved in the allocation of warden-controlled accommodation. Housing managers and occupational therapists work closely together to ensure that, through their knowledge of an individual's capabilities, special housing is properly allocated. They also provide care and support to elderly people in council accommodation. It is now quite common to discover occupational therapists advising housing departments on the necessary adaptations for handicapped tenants that need to be made to council houses – where rails should be, widths of doorways, turning space in rooms and corridors for wheelchairs. Where relatives are willing and able to accommodate the elderly, occupational therapists will be concerned with helping to make the house suitable for the elderly member of the family, particularly in ways which will facilitate independence and minimise the strain on the younger family.

The involvement of occupational therapy in the rehabilitation of the elderly in the various settings outlined does not necessarily lead to dramatic results or high discharge rates. The occupational therapist is in a team caring for the elderly, coping with many demands, enabling patients to enjoy a happy, dignified life in their old age. Where there is no occupational therapist available, information about suitable aids can be sought from the Disabled Living Foundation in Kensington, from Department of Health and Social Security Demonstration Centres, or by visiting local exhibitions of aids. The nearest hospital will give advice whenever they are able to do so, or will indicate the nearest occupational therapist or social worker who might assist.

11

NURSING CARE OF THE DYING

ALISON CHARLES-EDWARDS

formerly Ward Sister,
Michael Sobell House Continuing Care Unit, Oxford

The underlying aim of terminal care is to help people to die well, in comfort and with dignity. This can be achieved only if the needs of the body, mind and soul are met. It is essential to create an atmosphere in which adjustment to forthcoming death can be encouraged and helped, but this will be of little value if, meanwhile, severe pain is left untreated. Similarly, pain-relieving drugs will be less effective, however skilfully used, if they are prescribed in a cold and indifferent manner. The very highest standards of care may be achieved in vain, unless every aspect is tailored to the needs of the individual patient and family.

PATIENTS' ATTITUDES TO DEATH

Some elderly patients who become terminally ill welcome death. It may be that their present condition has been preceded by a long, painful illness, by a loss of independence, by loneliness after the death of a spouse, or they may have simply grown weary with life. Others, however, will display as much fighting spirit and determination to go on living as any 20-year-old. The majority show great ambivalence, saying that they are quite ready to die one minute, whilst worrying about any signs of deterioration the next. When caring for someone who is dying, it is always helpful to find out what his attitude is, in order to respond appropriately.

CARERS' ATTITUDES TO DEATH

Nowadays, many people reach middle age without encountering death at firsthand, unless they happen to work with the sick, or have seen active military service. Less than one death in three now occurs in the home, and it is no longer customary to take the body home to rest until the funeral. As unfamiliarity with death has increased, so has the fear which it produces. Every time we care for someone who is dying, we are forced, whether consciously or unconsciously, to acknowledge the fact that we and all our loved ones will also die one day. It is important to allow these feelings to surface and to work towards accepting death as an inevitable and wholly natural ending to life, rather than viewing it as a medical failure. Those who are overwhelmed by their own fear of death, and by their anger with the medical profession for failing to prevent it, will find it difficult to have a close relationship with someone who is dying. To avoid the feelings of fear and anger being aroused, the carer may, unknowingly, distance herself from the patient and his suffering, although the dying person will need the support of close relationships above all else.

THE MODE OF DYING

Most elderly people have a gentle, peaceful death, with minimal physical discomfort and little or no apparent mental anguish. In some, however, both mental and physical suffering may be severe, requiring a great deal of skilled help. Everything tends to happen more slowly in old age, including the progression of disease, and dying may be a very long, drawn-out process. This can be a rich and healing time, when families draw together, supporting each other in their grief, as they say their 'goodbyes', their 'sorrys' and their 'thank yous'. For others, the length and uncertainty of the last weeks can seem intolerable, particularly where one relative is providing most of the care single-handed. Neighbours and friends can make so much difference by offering to sit with the patient occasionally, by helping with the practical chores and by spending time listening to the relative's worries.

APPROPRIATE TREATMENT

There comes a time during most fatal illnesses when curative treatment is no longer appropriate. This may be because the side-effects are as distressing and life-endangering as the disease itself, because the treatment has proved ineffective, or because the patient's basic condition is such that any prolongation of his life would be meddlesome. These decisions are never easy or clear-cut and each case must be considered individually. The doctor will consult the family or close friends, the nursing staff and anyone else involved in the patient's care, but the patient's own wishes, if they can be ascertained, will always take precedence.

Almost everyone involved in caring for the aged will have witnessed situations where the wrong decision was made and inappropriate treatment was given. The following is an example of this.

> The patient was a man in his late 80s, who was severely demented. He had had two strokes and was no longer able to communicate. He had been in hospital for nine years and had been bed-bound for all that time. He lay permanently curled up in a foetal position, with his eyes closed. He was incontinent of urine and faeces, and had bed sores and severely contracted limbs, which were almost certainly painful. A nephew visited him about every six weeks. On developing a chest infection, instead of allowing nature to take its course, antibiotics were given by injection. He recovered from the chest infection, only to die of a urine infection six months later.

If a team approach is used, whereby doctors, nurses and relatives all pool their thinking, and reach a joint decision, this kind of situation will be avoided.

EMOTIONAL SUPPORT

Patients who are terminally ill are invariably aware that they are dying, whether or not they talk about it. This knowledge will arouse a turmoil of emotions.

Fear

There may be fear of suffering and pain which many elderly people, remembering scenes of death-bed agony, believe to be an inevitable part of dying. There may be fear of judgement and punishment in the next life, too, since this plays a major role in the faith of many older people. Like any other fear, the fear of dying is likely to be worse at night, when feelings of isolation are heightened. The darkness seems to magnify fear a hundredfold. In the familiarity of one's own home, especially if there is someone sleeping beside you, the fear may not be so intense. Nurses on night-duty need to be especially observant. Half an hour spent sitting with a patient, sharing his fears, is a much better use of time than serving up unlimited cups of tea. Reassuring a patient that almost all pain can now be relieved, that he will probably die in his sleep, and that he will not be left alone at the end, may do a great deal to alleviate his fears.

Grief

Even those who have led the most impoverished and lonely lives, will grieve in anticipation over the loss of someone or something that they love, as well as over life itself. The depth of grief can be immense when a spouse is still alive, or when a son or daughter, a close friend or grandchild are to be left.

Guilt

Guilt about pain caused to others, broken promises or family feuds, for example, may weigh heavily on the dying person's conscience, and there is often a great desire to 'make things right' before they die.

Anger

Even those who are in their 90s may experience great anger at having their lives curtailed before they are ready. Anger can be displaced on to those people with whom the patient feels safest and by whom he feels most loved and respected – usually close relatives, who will feel hurt and confused. They will need a great deal of support to help them to understand this behaviour, so that they do not retaliate or withdraw from the dying person when they are most needed.

Depression

Many elderly people have had years of disability, pain or loneli-ness before they die, so it is not surprising that depression is common amongst the terminally ill. People tend to look back critically over their lives when they are approaching death, examining their family life, their friendships, their marriages and their contribution to society. Some are disappointed and depressed by what they see. Those caring for them can help to focus their thoughts on their times of happiness and their achievements, and to find explanations for their failings.

Joy and relief

Many elderly people will feel great relief to know that the end of their suffering is in sight. Those with a firm faith in a life after death may anticipate their reunion with God (if Christian) and with their loved ones, with nothing but joy.

The most important role of those caring for the dying is to allow all these feelings to be shared. To make this possible, a relationship of safety and trust must be developed and the carer must learn to listen. Listening should not be seen as a passive activity. The quality of listening that is needed demands maximum attention and a willingness to experience what it feels like to be that dying person.

Nurses are always anxious to make people feel better and, if they see a patient looking sad, will instinctively try to cheer him up. But we should not expect dying patients to be constantly cheerful. If we see them looking sad, we should go and sit quietly beside them and make it clear that we are prepared to listen. If the patient begins to cry, we should encourage the tears, rather than try to stop them. Given this kind of support, the painful feelings may eventually lessen. By the time that they die, many elderly people seem to have reached a state of tranquillity and acceptance.

Most people appear to have spiritual needs of some kind, particularly those who are approaching death, whether or not they aspire to a specific faith and whether or not their needs are expressed in religious terms. The person providing pastoral care, whether a vicar, a priest, a rabbi, the next-door neighbour or a nurse, will need, first of all, to develop a relationship with the dying person, which enables the sharing of deep and often painful thoughts and feelings, and which offers help in dealing with them. All manner of spiritual concerns may need exploring together. These include discussion about man's purpose in life, life after death, euthanasia, the relationship between sin and suffering, and how to explain death to children and to prepare them for it. The carer should not struggle to answer these questions, because his or her answers may not help. The only relevant solutions are those which the dying person works out for himself.

For the dying patient who is a Christian, there are many forms of worship. These include the sacraments, in particular, confession and absolution, Holy Communion and the anointing of the sick. Some patients in hospital wish to participate in communal worship, but others prefer to hear Bible readings or prayers said at their bedside. These are unfamiliar to many people, however, and need to be offered sensitively. Even in the fulfilment of these more specific services, the presence of the priest is not essential, unless the sacraments are being administered. Lay parishioners who are particular friends of the dying person, should feel able to say prayers at a patient's bedside, and most nurses, Christian or agnostic, would feel happy to read a patient's favourite passage or psalm from the Bible to him when he is too weak to read for himself. It is often the task of the nurse to inform the appropriate minister of religion when someone is seriously ill and to enlist his help in supporting the patient and those close to him.

It can be harmful to ask a minister of religion for help just when a patient is dying. The appearance of an unfamiliar person, who has obviously been summoned because death is imminent, will seem sinister and frightening to many patients, especially if they are at all confused or if they have never practised the faith to which they are nominally ascribed. Involvement at the earliest possible stage is the obvious answer, not least because the patient is then able to decide for himself whether or not this is desirable.

Ministers of religion and representatives of religious communities have an invaluable role to play in the care of dying patients, but they can only fulfil this role if they are included in the caring team. It is vital that everyone involved works in a united way. Information should be shared freely and support extended to every member of the team. This includes, of course, the ministers of religion, who can become isolated otherwise.

SYMPTOM CONTROL

It is never true to say that there is nothing more that can be done, medically, for a dying person. The control of pain, and the many other common symptoms, demands enormous commitment and skill. There may be as many as eight or nine different symptoms to be treated and all will need reviewing continuously. The following are some of the more common ones, and those which cause greatest distress to relatives, as well as to the patients themselves.

Pain

Pain is commonly feared by the dying; however, even amongst those dying of cancer, which is often associated with painful death, one in three patients experiences nothing more than discomfort. Pain is generally less severe and easier to control in the elderly. Most people recognise the psychological aspect of pain. The same pain stimulus produces widely differing emotional responses – pain which seems quite tolerable to one person

will be overwhelming to another. It is very easy to fall into the
trap of passing moral judgements and of confusing a high pain
threshold with courage. It is not difficult to be sympathetic with a
brave, uncomplaining patient, but it is easy to be critical of those
who are intolerant of seemingly minor pains. To avoid this
temptation, it is essential to accept that pain is precisely what the
patient says it is, occurring when he says it occurs and hurting as
much as he says it hurts.

Several minor pains can be more demoralising than one severe
one. The combination of a sore mouth infected with 'thrush',
constipation, and a superficial bed sore, may cause more distress
than a compressed nerve. Seemingly minor pains should be
taken seriously always and treated as conscientiously as the more
severe ones.

Almost all pain can be relieved nowadays, and even that which
cannot be alleviated completely, can be brought within tolerable
limits. Several drugs may need to be used in varying combina-
tions, but there are always alternatives if one treatment fails. If
pain is particularly severe, or difficult to control, the family
doctor, or hospital consultant, may call in a specialist from the
local hospice for advice. We need no longer allow anyone to die in
pain, or accept this as unavoidable.

Pain experienced by the terminally ill is usually constant. To
keep it under control it will be necessary to give analgesics (pain-
killers) regularly – generally every four hours. Pain produces fear
– fear that the pain will get worse and worse until it is intolerable.
The fear in turn makes the pain worse. To break this vicious cycle
of pain and fear, an analgesic has to be found which will alleviate
the pain completely. This is given at regular intervals, before the
pain returns. If the medication is withheld until the pain recurs,
the fear will also return, worsening the pain and resulting in a
higher dose of the analgesic being needed to relieve it. Strong
pain-killers do make people sleepy at first, but they usually adjust
after a few days. Anxious relatives are often perturbed by this
drowsiness and withhold the medication, but this should be
discouraged, since the first goal is always to free the dying person
of pain.

Nausea and vomiting

Nausea and vomiting have many causes, such as a tumour or
very severe constipation which has blocked the bowel, radiotherapy, the use of certain anti-cancer and pain-killing drugs, or

raised pressure in the skull from a brain haemorrhage or tumour. The cause of the vomiting should be established so that the most suitable drug can be given. These drugs are known as anti-emetics. The carer can also provide great support by placing a hand firmly on the patient's forehead during vomiting, and, afterwards, by providing a refreshing mouthwash, a warm, soapy flannel and towel, and a change of bed linen and night clothes, if these have been soiled.

Constipation

Constipation may be caused by the low intake of bulk food, weak, lax muscles, inactivity, paraplegia and the use of tranquillising and pain-killing drugs. Encouragement to eat foods with a high-fibre content, such as fruit, vegetables and whole grain cereals, plus an increase in the amount of fluids taken may be effective, but often an aperient will be necessary. The most useful ones are those which have two modes of action – they soften and increase the bulk of the bowel contents, whilst stimulating the muscular activity of the bowel. If the bowel tone is inadequate, regular suppositories or enemas may be necessary, but these should be avoided whenever possible.

Diarrhoea

Diarrhoea occurs less frequently. Although it can be treated quite easily with constipating drugs, such as codeine, care must be taken to ensure that the diarrhoea is not just an overflow from a bowel blocked with faeces.

Breathlessness

Breathlessness or dyspnoea can be a very frightening and exhausting symptom. To sit with someone fighting to breathe, and being unable to do anything to help, is a terrible experience which haunts many relatives long after the patient has died. A great deal of time will need to be spent in rearranging pillows and lifting the patient up in the bed, so that an upright position can be maintained in order to allow maximum expansion of the lungs. A foot-board or bolster at the bottom of the bed will help to prevent the patient from slipping down. Sitting in a chair may be the most comfortable position, even at night. A cool, circulating atmo-sphere is essential and, in warm weather, air conditioning and fans are a great help. Morphine-type drugs are the most useful in this instance, because they slow down the respiratory rate and alleviate anxiety. (They would not be suitable for breathless patients who are not terminally ill, however.)

Haemorrhage

Few symptoms cause more alarm to patients and relatives than the sight of blood. This is due to the horrifying appearance of even the smallest quantity, and its tendency to spread rapidly, making it look far more than it really is. Adrenaline can be used to stop the bleeding of surface lesions, and drugs are available which reduce haemorrhaging into the bladder or uterus. Patients and relatives need encouragement to share their fears about haemorrhaging, and it is often possible to reassure them that it does not represent any serious threat. Haemorrhage from a major artery is not common, and, when it does occur, although it is devastating for relatives to witness, it usually brings about a very quick, painless and peaceful death.

Dehydration

The terminally ill frequently become dehydrated, but the only symptom of any consequence resulting from this is a dry, uncomfortable mouth. Dry mouths rapidly become furred and dirty, and dirty mouths rapidly become infected, especially with thrush. Small quantities of fluid should be offered regularly, especially acidic drinks such as the juice of citrus fruits, lime or peppermint cordial, tonic or soda water, beer and tea, as these stimulate the secretion of saliva. Fruit jellies, chunks of fresh pineapple, acid drops and crushed ice are also useful in keeping the mouth moist. Regular teeth-cleaning and mouth-washes should be encouraged for as long as the patient can cope with them. When this is no longer possible, the carer can wrap a piece of gauze around her forefinger, dip it in a mouth-wash solution and gently clean the mouth. If the tongue is very furred, a little bicarbonate of soda, dissolved in warm water, will help to clean it.

Malodours

Malodours from infected lesions, from incontinence or from fistulae (which are openings leading out from the bowel), cause great mental anguish. Carers often find it hard to conceal their disgust, and the patient feels ashamed and alienated. Frequent washing with soap and water, thorough drying, and a change of night clothes and bed linen, is the best treatment. In addition, there are various substances which can be used, e.g. glycerine and thymol mouth-washes and chlorophyll tablets for bad breath, and special solutions for sprinkling on dressing pads, on bed linen or into colostomy bags, and the use of yoghurt and charcoal pads for dressings. Air-fresheners, cologne, sweet-smelling soap and talcum powder all have their use. Attempts to drown an unpleasant smell with a pleasant one can produce an even worse one, however, so caution is necessary.

Difficulty in swallowing

Difficulty in swallowing, or dysphagia, is not uncommon in those dying from neurological degenerative diseases, such as muscular dystrophy and motor-neurone disease. Great calmness and understanding is required, and, if the patient needs feeding, tiny amounts must be given very slowly. Liquidized food, or proprietary products such as Complan and Clinifeed, may be useful. Drugs offer no help in treating dysphagia.

These are just a few of the many symptoms that afflict the terminally ill. All need a combination of medication plus understanding, reassurance and skilled practical nursing.

CARING FOR THE DYING PERSON

Most elderly people prefer to die in their own bed at home, but this is not always possible, as it depends largely on the family's willingness and availability to help care for them. Some elderly people change their minds as they grow weaker, either wanting the security of qualified staff at hand, or feeling concern about the burden that they are to their families.

When patients are cared for in their own, or a relative's, home, they are often cared for extremely well, but are left very much alone between meals and bathtimes. Keeping the patient confined to his bedroom, and spending the minimum amount of time with him, is another example of how we can distance ourselves from the dying, if we have not come to terms with death. The patient feels lonely and isolated, unable to share his fears with anyone. He usually prefers to have his bed taken into the living room, where he can be part of family life.

When people are dying, they often feel that they are losing control of themselves and their lives. In hospital, it is particularly important that nursing care is performed at the patient's own pace, always explaining procedures slowly and clearly before they are performed. It is no longer appropriate to chivvy them to do things for themselves, but even when washing dying patients, or changing their wet beds, they should always be spoken to with great respect. Dying patients are often very emaciated and need handling with extreme gentleness. Food and drinks should be offered in very small quantities, and, if these are refused, there is no justification for trying to force them. This can easily become a source of great distress and guilt.

Most physical nursing care required by a dying patient, such as basic hygiene, mouth care, pressure area care and the management of the bowels, for example, is identical to the care needed by any elderly sick or bed-bound person, as described in the course of this book. The following case study shows how closely the physical and emotional aspects of care are entwined. The intimacy which develops between someone who is incapacitated by illness, and the person caring for them, is unique. Such a high level of security can be experienced when being blanket bathed or shaved, for example, that these are the times when the most painful questions may be asked and the deepest fears shared.

Mrs A was 92 when she died. She had first noticed the lump in her breast 19 years earlier. Several reasons seemed to have influenced her decision not to see her doctor about it. She had assumed from the outset that it was cancer, and knew that the treatments available, such as surgery or radiotherapy, were unpleasant. She also believed, quite mistakenly, that all cancer was incurable. The fact that she had nursed her own mother when she was dying of breast cancer, long before present treatments were developed, must have had a strong influence on her response.

Mrs A's husband had died less than one year previously, so she was feeling extremely lonely and bereft. This not only made the possibility of an early death seem less dreadful, but also (because she now lived alone) made it easy to conceal the lump. Since it was not painful, she was able to put it out of her mind for much of the time. Mrs A had no children, her closest relatives being a nephew and niece, both of whom were married with young families. One lived about 15 miles away and visited every two or three weeks.

To her surprise, the lump remained apparently unchanged for about 16 years, but it then began to grow quite suddenly and became painful. She took aspirins to dull the pain and, when it began to weep, padded it with old sheeting, but still told no one.

It was almost two years later when Mrs A's general practitioner was contacted by her niece who was concerned about a deterioration in her aunt's general condition and about the very unpleasant smell, which seemed worse each time she visited. The doctor visited Mrs A and discovered that she had advanced cancer of the breast which had broken through to the surface skin so that a massive ulcerated area now covered her upper chest. Secondary growths had infiltrated her lungs, so she was extremely breathless and weak. As the ulcerated area was so soggy and bled easily, the doctor persuaded Mrs A to have a short course of radiotherapy to help dry the area, prevent bleeding and to make it less offensive and more manageable.

During the five days that she was in hospital, the health visitor arranged for Mrs A to have meals on wheels on her return, for a home help to call on her five days a week, for a supply of incontinence sheets to be delivered, plus the special incineration bags for their disposal, and for the local 'Good Neighbour' scheme to send a visitor in each day to do shopping and any other necessary jobs. This was first approved by Mrs A and then by her niece, whom the health visitor met when visiting Mrs A in hospital. By this time Mrs A was feeling so wretched that she willingly accepted any help that was offered.

On her return from hospital, the district nursing sister began visiting twice daily to provide general nursing care and to dress the breast lesion. They soon discovered that the best way to do the dressing was to remove the outer layers of padding and then to help Mrs A into a warm saline bath (one teacupful of salt added to the water). They would leave her to soak for 5 to 10 minutes whilst making the bed and preparing the sterile dressing pack. In this way the inner layers of the dressing could be lifted without removing any newly healed skin and without causing bleeding or pain. The shower attachment was used to cleanse the lesion, but care was taken to get the temperature to blood heat and to keep the water pressure low. Paraffin gauze was used to prevent sticking, and both yoghurt and charcoal pads were applied to reduce malodours.

This procedure was carried out every morning, which made it easy to keep an eye on the condition of pressure areas and to massage arachis oil into the skin when it became dry and flaky. Only the outer layers of the dressing were renewed at the evening visit. Mrs A felt embarrassed and degraded by the terrible appearance and smell of the lesion, but the twice daily dressing reduced these problems, and the nurses were careful never to show any sign of revulsion when removing the soiled dressings.

Mrs A was now admitting to a great deal of pain, but this was quite easily controlled with a small dose (10 mg) of oral morphine in a liquid solution, which she took faithfully every four hours. Unfortunately, the morphine did cause constipation so a daily aperient was also necessary. The nurses observed the efficacy of both these medications with care, reporting to the doctor whenever they felt an adjustment of the dose was called for.

Although reserved at first, Mrs A soon got to know her nurses and seemed to look forward to their visits. Whenever they could, they would sit with her for a while and encourage her to talk. She was stoical and totally uncomplaining, but, after a few weeks, she felt secure enough to ask one of the nurses what was likely to happen over the next few weeks and how she would die, and to share her great fear of haemorrhaging.

The nurse explained honestly and gently that the most likely sequence of events would be that she would gradually get weaker until she would not feel like getting up any more. She would then become sleepy, gradually sleeping for more and more of the day. She would eventually go into a deeper sleep during which her breathing would get slower and slower until it stopped altogether and she died. The nurse was able to tell her that a haemorrhage was extremely unlikely and to reassure her that, if it did happen, loss of consciousness would be so fast that she would hardly know anything about it. Mrs A found this enormously comforting as she had terrible fears of being racked with pain at the moment of death.

Mrs A had often expressed her desire to die at home and not to go into hospital. Fortunately, her niece was able to stay with her once she became bedbound. Five days after that she died, very peacefully.

Many people imagine that terminal care must be very depressing, but in reality it can be enormously satisfying work. The privilege of helping someone to end his life in comfort, the depth of the relationships which so often develop between the dying and those caring for them, and the close bonds which form within a team engaged in this work, are just three of the reasons why this is so.

Further reading

Charles-Edwards, Alison, *The Nursing Care of the Dying Patient* (Beaconsfield Publishers Ltd, 1983).

Kübler–Ross, Elizabeth, *On Death and Dying* (Tavistock Publications, 1973).

Lamerton, Richard, *Care of the Dying* (Penguin, 1980).

12

A HELPING HAND

PAT YOUNG
Editor-in-Chief, Geriatric Medicine

It is useful for a nurse to know something about the various organisations that offer practical help and support to the sick, disabled elderly and those who care for them. Gaps do occur in the services provided by the State, and there are a number of voluntary charitable organisations that do a sterling job in filling those gaps. In addition, the 'private sector' in medical and nursing care has much to offer, and it is not necessarily beyond everyone's means.

First of all, one must have some understanding of what Social Service Departments have to offer. They do not come under the National Health Service, but are run by the local authorities; many people think that this separation of the health service from the social services is not particularly helpful. It would certainly seem more logical, from the organisational point of view, if they were much more closely integrated.

You will have read in chapter 10 that many Social Service Departments have an occupational therapist on the staff, whose job it is to visit patients' homes, often when they are still in hospital, to see how easy it will be for them to manage their daily lives, if they have a disability resulting from their illness, and to see whether any aids or adaptations to the home will be needed to help them perform such routine activities as getting in and out of the bath, on and off the toilet, or up and down stairs.

Social Service Departments are mainly responsible for providing services, such as home helps, meals on wheels, lunch clubs and day centres, and laundry services. In addition they provide aids for daily living, organise house alterations, install telephones and pay their rental, supply radio and television sets, and license them. Their full range of responsibilities is laid down in the Chronically Sick and Disabled Persons Act 1970, under which they should provide virtually any service that a handicapped person requires in order to enable him or her to lead an independent life. However, there are not always sufficient funds available to provide the full range, and this is where the voluntary organisations have an important part to play.

Social Service Departments are staffed mainly by social workers, some of whom specialise in working with elderly people. Their job is a delicate one, demanding great tact, patience and perseverance, and a comprehensive knowledge of all the local resources. They visit their 'clients' at home, in order to assess their background, life style, family relationships and needs, and have to be able to discuss such matters as personal finances, in order that they can assess how much the client can afford to pay, and how much assistance he or she will need. It may be possible to maintain an elderly person at home by supplying a home help twice a week, with meals on wheels every day, if the client can't get out and about; or with regular visits to a day centre for a daily meal, social contacts and activities. The time may have come, however, when the old person is unable to cope at home, even with such support, and the social worker may then recommend that he goes either into 'sheltered accommodation' (a warden-supervised flat, for instance) or a residential home. However incapacitated, an old person will be very loath to leave his own home, so the social worker will have to deal with this situation with great tact and sensitivity.

Departments of Social Service maintain records of all sources of help and types of accommodation for the elderly, and work closely with the voluntary and charitable organisations in their areas, so that the client is given the full range of options and can choose according to his means and background. For instance, a number of organisations, such as Age Concern, Help the Aged, the British Legion, and other similar bodies, have housing schemes in various parts of the country which the client may consider preferable to a local authority residential home.

Of the various organisations concerned with the welfare of the elderly, Age Concern is the oldest and largest. It has four national bodies, one for each country in the United Kingdom, and over 1,300 autonomous local groups, each providing direct services for the old in its locality. Housing is a top priority and Age Concern groups run, or help to run, homes for the elderly. They form housing associations to provide sheltered accommodation, offer a housing advisory service for old people and their relatives, support the elderly who want to stay in their own homes, and campaign for laws relating to housing to be improved.

Another top priority is health, and here Age Concern offers help which is eminently practical, in the form of stroke clubs, day centres for the physically disabled, special centres for the elderly mentally infirm, hospital after-care support schemes, and short-stay convalescent homes. It lends equipment such as wheelchairs, campaigns for improved domiciliary services of all kinds, and provides hearing advice bureaux that check hearing aids and advise on the different types available.

Transport is another of Age Concern's projects. It provides minibuses (to take the elderly to and from day centres), lunch clubs and clinics, as well as car services to enable them to visit relatives or their family doctor, or to go shopping. One imaginative group operates a 'Cuppa-Caravan' scheme – a mobile club which visits villages in remote country districts with no social amenities, to serve coffee and tea, carry large-print library books and act as an advice and information service. There is, in fact, no need which Age Concern leaves unfulfilled, and it is always worth contacting your local group when you need help. The address and telephone number will be listed in your local telephone directory.

Help the Aged is the other big charitable organisation concerned with the health and welfare of the elderly. It is chiefly a campaigning and fund-raising body, and there are Help the Aged gift shops in most major shopping centres which provide a continuous flow of funds towards the help so badly needed. Housing is a top priority with this organisation, too, and Help the Aged has its own housing association in the United Kingdom, with schemes for sheltered accommodation and residential homes all over the country. It supports and provides funds for medical projects great and small, ranging from building and equipping rehabilitation units, to buying items of equipment for a mobile physiotherapy unit. The policy is to give help where there is obvious enterprise and initiative, and a worth-while project to support.

Help and advice of a more immediately practical nature is also available from the British Red Cross Society, the St John Ambulance Association and Brigade, its Scottish equivalent – the St Andrew's Ambulance Association – and the Women's Royal

Voluntary Service. For addresses of these organisations, see page 172.

The British Red Cross Society (BRCS) is part of the International Red Cross movement and one of the 130 National Red Cross Societies. There are seven principles of the Red Cross: humanity, impartiality, neutrality, independence, voluntary service, unity and universality. The primary purpose is protection for sick and wounded victims of war – the Red Cross is the emblem of the medical services of the armed forces. In peacetime, the Red Cross Societies – one in each country – work to alleviate suffering among the sick, the injured, the disabled and the frail elderly. The BRCS trains its members and members of the public in first aid, home nursing and associated subjects, and provides a wide range of services. It is a voluntary organisation, relying on public support, and is governed by a council and managed by trustees. It has branches all over the country, whose addresses can be found in the local telephone directory. The services provided for the local community include first aid duties at public and sporting events, nursing visits to patients' homes under the supervision of a district nursing sister, help at health centres, group practices, foot clinics and blood transfusion donor centres, escorting sick and elderly people on journeys, and helping at clubs and day centres, and at holidays and play groups for handicapped children.

The work of the BRCS in hospital is invaluable, ranging from simple nursing duties, to running shops and library services, and giving beauty care. Perhaps less well known is the support it gives to the frail elderly being nursed at home. For instance, it will supply (on loan) medical equipment such as wheelchairs, arrange for members to sit in with patients to relieve the strain on the family, perform such routine chores as shopping, changing library books, hair washing, or drop in for a friendly chat, providing understanding and sympathetic support in difficult, stressful situations. Red Cross members often use their own cars to supply transport for the elderly, they run the meals on wheels service in some areas for the local authority, and they organise stroke clubs, hearing circles for the deaf, social clubs and day centres, as well as group holidays at suitable venues where Red Cross members care for the guests throughout their stay, giving their relatives an opportunity to take a holiday themselves. They also provide an important link between hospital and home, visiting patients before discharge to see what help may be needed when they return home, and to see that the house is aired, the bed ready, and enough food available if they live alone. The BRCS can be regarded as a lifeline, both for aged patients and for those nursing them, and it is well worth contacting your local branch for help in time of need.

Similar organisations are the St John Ambulance Association and Brigade in England, and the St Andrew's Ambulance Association in Scotland. These two bodies are perhaps best known for providing first aid at public events of all kinds, from a local soccer match to a royal wedding. In addition, they carry out nursing duties in hospitals and in patients' homes, and take a special interest in the welfare of the elderly.

The Order of St John of Jerusalem dates from the time of the crusades when the brothers tended pilgrims on their way to Jerusalem. The Ambulance Association is one of its three great foundations, and is responsible for training; another foundation is the Brigade, whose uniforms are so familiar at public functions. Both members and cadets of the St John Ambulance serve the elderly population in their local divisions in much the same way as BRCS members – doing nursing duties in hospitals and in patients' homes, helping with transport, doing the shopping, taking in meals, arranging diversionary activities, such as outings, clubs and coffee mornings, organising meals for festive occasions, such as Christmas and birthdays, and providing a 'granny sitting' service and overnight supervision. The cadets, in particular, have an excellent rapport with the elderly, visiting them, reading to them, shopping for them, exercising their pets and doing their gardening and any other tasks.

The St Andrew's Ambulance Association came into existence just over 100 years ago, in Glasgow, which was then a rapidly expanding industrial city with – even then – a traffic problem. As there were so many road and industrial accidents, the overworked local doctors and nurses needed help. By the end of the first year, 500 volunteer members of the Association had been trained in first aid, in order to cope with the crisis. Now the Association has a membership of well over 20,000, plus 2,000 cadets, and its uniformed Ambulance Corps carry out a full range of first aid duties and support services for the sick and elderly throughout Scotland.

These three organisations have combined to produce an excellent nursing manual, written by the Chief Nursing Officer of the St John Ambulance Association and Brigade, called *Caring for the*

Sick. It is aimed at those without any training who need simple, practical guidance and instruction in the basic nursing procedures. Of course, all three bodies also provide excellent training courses in first aid and home nursing.

Another voluntary organisation which provides invaluable practical support is the Women's Royal Voluntary Service (WRVS). Formed in 1938 by the Dowager Marchioness of Reading, at the request of the Home Secretary, to recruit women to help with air raid precautions, this service undertook clothing, feeding and billeting evacuee children and their parents, as well as many other wartime duties, such as running canteens for servicemen. Nowadays it continues its service to the community in many different ways, with help for the elderly figuring largely in its welfare work. It is responsible, for instance, for over 2,000 social clubs throughout Great Britain where the old can meet in a friendly atmosphere, entertain themselves with films, talks, games and sing-songs, and generally enjoy social contacts and activities. There are also luncheon clubs and all-day clubs for the isolated and lonely, some with chiropody clinics. WRVS members also drive old people to these clubs, so that they don't become housebound.

For those unable to get out and about, WRVS operate the meals on wheels service for the local authority and keep a friendly and unobtrusive eye on the people they visit in case they need more help. They organise home visits and help with domestic chores, such as shopping, gardening and decorating; run 'Good Neighbour' schemes; provide books on wheels from a mobile library; provide support in the home when an old person is discharged from hospital; and work closely with the local police, who call on them for help in times of crisis. In addition to all this, the WRVS has a housing association which converts old houses into flats and flatlets for the elderly. These have resident caretakers. It runs 22 residential clubs, one 'extra-care' club and one nursing home. There are local WRVS offices in all parts of the country, which provide a similar range of services to that of the other voluntary organisations. The addresses of local offices are in the telephone directory; further information can be obtained from the WRVS London headquarters (address on page 172).

An organisation which offers a useful service not directly to the old, but to all professions engaged in caring for the sick and handicapped, is the Disabled Living Foundation. It has an aids centre at its London headquarters (address on page 172), where nurses and others can see the full range of practical equipment their patients may need – from wheelchairs to incontinence pads – and get expert advice from the qualified staff on the respective advantages of aids and their suitability for individual patients. There is also a comprehensive information service on all aspects of disability, as well as a reference library containing books, pamphlets, current periodicals, with reading lists on such specialised topics as strokes and design for the disabled and the elderly disabled. The DLF has produced a number of useful publications on such subjects as incontinence equipment and clothing, and foot care for the elderly and disabled, and offers an advisory service on these and other relevant topics, such as chronic skin conditions, visual impairment, physical recreation and gardening for the disabled, and music therapy. Anyone caring for the elderly would find this organisation a valuable source of advice and information.

There are, of course, a number of other organisations concerned with specific diseases, such as multiple sclerosis, Parkinson's disease, chest, heart, and stroke problems, and so on, which give advice and support to sufferers and those who care for them. In the field of cancer, there are two bodies which perhaps deserve special mention: the Marie Curie Memorial Foundation and the National Society for Cancer Relief, both of which provide nursing homes and nursing services specialising in care of the cancer patient and care of the dying. (See page 172 for the addresses of these two organisations.)

We must not forget the many excellent privately-run residential and nursing homes, as well as the nursing agencies which supply trained nursing and care staff to give home nursing help. Some of these are run by commercial companies and some by charitable organisations; all should be licensed by the health or local authority, who inspect them regularly and maintain records of those in their respective areas.

It is good to know that there are so many people and organisations putting so much effort into helping the most vulnerable groups in society today. It shows that we do care about our fellow human beings, that we want to give them practical help in times of need or distress, and that we are willing to put ourselves out to do so. The voluntary movement is obviously strong and thriving in Britain, offering help and support where and how it is most needed. It is good to be able to end this book on such a positive and hopeful note.

Some useful addresses

Age Concern (England)
Bernard Sunley House
60 Pitcairn Road
Mitcham
Surrey CR4 3LL
(Telephone: 01-640 5431)
The British Red Cross Society
9 Grosvenor Crescent
London SW1X 7EJ
(Telephone: 01-235 5454)
Disabled Living Foundation
346 Kensington High Street
London W14 8NS
(Telephone: 01-602 2491)
Help the Aged
St James's Walk
London EC1R 0BE
(Telephone: 01-253 0253)
Marie Curie Memorial Foundation
28 Belgrave Square
London SW1X 8QG
(Telephone: 01-235 3325)
National Society for Cancer Relief
Michael Sobell House
30 Dorset Square
London NW1 6QL
(Telephone: 01-402 8125)
St John Ambulance
1 Grosvenor Crescent
London SW1X 7EF
(Telephone: 01-235 5231)
St Andrew's Ambulance Association
Milton Street
Glasgow G4
(Telephone: 041-332 4031)
Women's Royal Voluntary Service
17 Old Park Lane
London W1Y 4AJ
(Telephone: 01-499 6040)

INDEX

functional assessment, 144
functional disorders, 38–42

glaucoma, 15, 101–102
grooming, xvi, 74–80

haemorrhage, 160
  cerebral, 18, 103
hair, xiii, 2, 75, 78
handicap, physical, 16–24, 36
handling patients, 132–35
health and nutrition, 43–44
hearing, 33, 99–101
  aids, 13, 14; and communication, 100
heart, 21–24
  block, 7; digoxin, 54–5; disease,
    21–24; failure, 22; rate, 6–7
heating, 89, 90
Help the Aged, 166, 172
hip, osteoarthritis, 20
home:
  adaptations to, 143, 151; assessment
    of, 139–40, 141; 165; care, 95; living
    alone at, 95, 145, 166; rehabilita-
    tion, 126–29
hospitals, 92–3, 141, 142
  admission to, 98–99, 143; equip-
    ment, 143
housing, 151, 166–67, 170
hypertension, 4, 22, 54
hypnotics, 52–53
hypomania, 38–40, 41
hypotension, 4–5
hypothermia, 5–6

illness 4, 43–4
  psychiatric, 34–43; terminal, 46,
    152–64
impaction, 73
incontinence, xiii–xv, 69–72, 85–6
  faecal, 73; origins, 26–27; and
    physiotherapy, 119–21; stress-
    induced, 141
infection, 12
information, 171
ischaemia of limbs, 23

joints:
  diseases, 20; inflammation, 16–17

Korsakoff's psychosis, 44

late paraphrenia, 41–42
laxatives, 53–54

legs:
  broken, 117; circulation, 23; 'rest-
    less', 13; ulcers, 23–24
lifting, 134–45, 136
lighting, 89, 90
limbs, ischaemia of, 23
loneliness, 94, 107

Marie Curie Memorial Foundation,
  171, 172
meals on wheels, 90, 110–12
medicines, see drugs
memory failure, 31, 33, 35–36, 37
  assessing, 38, 39; and depression,
    40–1; Korsakoff's psychosis, 44
Ménière's disease, 14, 100–101
mental condition, 85
mental illness, 28–47
  classification, 35; occupational ther-
    apy, 145–47
menu planning, 114–15
mobility, xii, 85, 117–37
mood disturbances, 38–41
morphine, 56–57
mouth care, 63, 78–79, 160–61

nails, 2, 75
National Society for Cancer Relief, 171,
  172
nervous system, 17–20
neurotic disorders, 34, 42–43
nursing, 11, 59–87
  bad, x; of the dying, 152–64; process,
    59
nursing agencies, 171
nutrition, see diet and nutrition

occupational therapy, 138–51
  assessment, 143–44; in community,
    148–51; in continuing care, 148;
    home assessment, 139–40, 141,
    165; for mentally ill, 145–47
Order of St John of Jerusalem, 169–70
organisations, helpful, 165–71
osteoarthritis, 20
osteomalacia, 112

pain:
  in the dying, 56–57, 152, 157–58;
    drugs for, 55–56; and sleep, 82–83
Parkinson's disease, 19–20, 54
personality, and neurotic disorders,
  42–43
pets, 94, 108